EXPECTED
MIRACLES

EXPECTED MIRACLES

Surgeons at Work

Joan Cassell

TEMPLE UNIVERSITY PRESS ✳ *Philadelphia*

Temple University Press, Philadelphia 19122
Copyright © 1991 by Joan Cassell. All rights reserved
Published 1991
Printed in the United States of America

The paper used in this publication meets the minimum
requirements of American National Standard for Information
Sciences—Permanence of Paper for Printed Library Materials,
ANSI Z39.48-1984 ∞

Library of Congress Cataloging-in-Publication Data
Cassell, Joan.
Expected miracles : surgeons at work / Joan Cassell.
p.   cm.
Includes bibliographical references and index.
ISBN 0-87722-804-3 cloth
ISBN 0-87722-838-8 paper
1. Surgeons.   2. Surgeons—Attitudes.   I. Title.
RD31.5.C37   1991
617'.0232—dc20   90-43859
                                                  CIP

Epigraph on page 9 from "East Coker" in *Four Quartets*, copyright 1943 by
T. S. Eliot and renewed 1971 by Esme Valerie Eliot, reprinted by permission
of Harcourt Brace Jovanovich, Inc.

"The Good Surgeon: Colleagues' Evaluations" in Chapter 1 is adapted from
Joan Cassell, "The Good Surgeon," *International Journal of Moral and Social
Studies* 2, no. 2 (Summer 1987):155–71. Copyright © 1987 by Journals Ltd.

Chapter 2, "The Temperament of Surgeons," is adapted from Joan Cassell, "Of
Control, Certitude and the 'Paranoia' of Surgeons," *Culture, Medicine and Psy-
chiatry* 11, no. 2 (1987):229–49, © 1987 by D. Reidel Publishing Company,
reprinted by permission of Kluwer Academic Publishers, and Joan Cassell,
"Dismembering the Image of God: Surgeons, Wimps, Heroes and Miracles,"
Anthropology Today 2, no. 2 (1986):13–16.

Chapter 3, "The Fellowship of Surgeons," is adapted from Joan Cassell, "The
Fellowship of Surgeons, the Morality Play, and Social Control," *International
Journal of Moral and Social Studies* 4, no. 3 (Autumn 1989):195–212. Copyright
© 1989 by Journals Ltd.

Epigraph on page 219 from "Little Gidding" in *Four Quartets*, copyright 1943
by T. S. Eliot and renewed 1971 by Esme Valerie Eliot, reprinted by permission
of Harcourt Brace Jovanovich, Inc.

For M. W.

He knows why.

Non ridere, non lugere, neque detestari, sed intelligere.

(Not to ridicule, not to deplore, not to denounce, but to understand.)

Spinoza (*Ethica*)

CONTENTS

CAST OF CHARACTERS

Dr. Johnston, an Exemplary Surgeon:

"He has good academics, good background, looks the role, has good technical ability, takes care of the folks." (colleague)

Dr. Verdi, an Exemplary (and Paranoid) Surgeon:

"The whole damn world's against me!"

Dr. Bryna, a Compassionate Young Surgeon:

"He possesses all those qualities you wish for in your doctor—concern, compassion, confidence, and just a general T.L.C. manner." (patient)

Dr. Auerbach, a Sleazy Surgeon:

"Unfortunately, he has more woof than warp." (assistant chief of surgery)

Dr. Sylva, an Old-Time Prima Donna:

"You lay it down in their language and give them the confidence that you're the best thing that ever happened to them. It's like making love to a woman!"

Dr. Sutton, a Buffoon:

"He just does not know or is too proud to call for help

when he needs it. He's had more complications in a year than any surgeon I know." (colleague)

Raoul, a Prima Donna Chief Resident:

"Another miracle!"

The Setting:

The surgeons perform their morality play in a generic teaching hospital. If not quite Everyhospital, it resembles similar institutions throughout the United States. For legal, ethical, and traditional anthropological reasons, identifying details have been intentionally confused: locations are blurred, cases altered, minor characters merged. (See pages 223–25 for a description of the research sample and process.)

PREFACE

Some Words for Social Scientists

Le style c'est l'homme même.

George-Louis Leclerc de Buffon
Discours sur le Style

The way of saying is the what of saying.

Clifford Geertz
Works and Lives: The Anthropologist as Author

In this preface, I address my professional colleagues in order to explain why I have refrained from doing so in the remainder of the book. The lay reader who finds social scientific disputation tedious may happily ignore this section and skip to the introduction. (The interested non–social scientist might find it helpful to read the brief description of "ethnography" on pages 227–28.)[1]

I begin by taking exception to a prevalent genre in which the social scientist takes a position of moral superiority vis-à-vis the powerful people she has studied. Then, I address some issues that have been much discussed recently, such as authorial voice, reflexivity, and the positioned subject,[2] and other issues that have been invoked with less frequency, such as "the ways in which anthropology [and sociology] texts are written so as to exclude all but the committed fellow professional from the exclusive circle of understanding."[3]

xiii

THE ETHNOGRAPHY OF INDIGNATION

One of the rewards of deep thought is the hot glow of
anger at discovering a wrong.

Jules Henry
Pathways to Madness

At a professional meeting some years ago I met a colleague
who had spent several years doing fieldwork in hospitals.
When she learned that I had been funded to study the morality
of surgeons, she assumed without question that I was inves-
tigating their *immorality*. Suggesting I read an article on how
butchers keep their self-esteem despite their defiling profession, she said, laughingly, of surgeons: "They're all butchers,
really! I don't know how they can go home after their work,"
adding, in a contemptuous tone, "They're not really doctors!"

This social scientist, like many of my colleagues, adopted
an unthinking attitude of moral superiority to the powerful
people she had studied. Why did she feel superior? Is this
woman more moral, more scrupulous, more caring than the
doctors we both observed? (I know her and doubt this.) Is
the morality of social scientists superior to that of the powerful groups we, on occasion, study—and, on more occasions,
criticize?

Framed this way, the answer is so obvious that I seem to
be creating a straw man just to demolish it. But the issue is not
simple. My questions cover a tangle of unexamined attitudes,
emotions, and motives. If we make the rational assumption
that doctors, and other powerful people, probably exhibit the
same statistical distribution of goodness and evil as the rest of
the population—including social scientists—the query about
the assumed moral superiority of social scientists remains. It
is true that the powerful have the capacity to do more harm
than those with less power. This does not, however, explain
the automatic and unthinking assumption of evil.

There are reasons why social scientists might assume bad faith on the part of the powerful, feel superior, and then cast themselves as the scourges of God, whose self-appointed task is to cast out the money changers from the temple.

First, we must remember that identification with the victim, with its consequent anger against victimizers, is a traditional ethnographic stance. The social scientist who studies exotic, deviant, poor, and powerless peoples perceives adversity, suffering, and exploitation. As a representative of a more powerful society, the ethnographer may feel guilt as well as sympathy. Many of us become advocates for the peoples we study. In such cases, sympathy, empathy, and identification with powerless and victimized peoples is taken for granted as the "natural" behavior of any perceptive, feeling person. Identification with the victim is considered so legitimate, necessary, and morally admirable that it is accepted without question, even when an ethnographer's research does not concern victims.

Since field-workers who study the powerless seem to have nothing to gain from identifying with such peoples and taking their side against the powerful, colleagues assume they are ignoring self-interest in order to advance the interests of oppressed, despised, and subjugated groups. These critics tend to overlook the position of the observer, proceeding as though the researcher were transparent, occupying no specific role with its own structure of rules and rewards. Such naïveté is interesting on the part of social scientists. Such critics proceed as though the concepts and techniques of social science were designed solely to examine and record the Other (the passive one who is studied rather than the active one who studies) and assume that the observer who investigates and identifies with deviant and powerless groups is (or should be) immune to critical observation.

When we examine the social and professional rules and rewards that affect field-workers, we discover that in academic life, where most are located, rewards do indeed exist for empathizing with and championing (rather than blaming) the victim.

We find interactive rewards: studying people less powerful than oneself is more emotionally and socially (if not physically) comfortable than studying those with more power, even if that comfort involves merely people's tolerating one's presence. The field-worker possesses social power compared with those studied, and if this powerful researcher takes the role of advocate, group members may well be grateful.

Academic rewards exist as well: becoming a specialist in and symbolic member of a little-known deviant or powerless group gives one one's own little portion of academic "turf," to be discussed with colleagues, imparted to students, and displayed in articles and monographs.

The imputation of virtue, by oneself and one's colleagues, for justifying and supporting the "victims," is also rewarding. Defender of the powerless is a comfortable moral position to adopt.

I am in no way suggesting it is morally questionable or disreputable for a field-worker to identify with and protect powerless groups. Such field-workers are not necessarily self-sacrificing, however, and an attitude of righteousness—if indeed they exhibit one—may be unjustified.

Many ethnographers expand their mandate to exalt the humble to a related injunction to put down the mighty. The imputation of virtue by oneself and others for defending the victim is then extended to attacking the victimizers. Here we encounter the ethnographer as neo-Marxist prophet, doing the Lord's work. Burning with the hot glow of anger, the field-worker assails the powerful and censures colleagues who do not go and do likewise. Unlike Jesus, however, who cautioned about casting the first stone, the ethnographer of indignation is profoundly self-righteous.

There's no getting around it—burning with the hot glow of

anger feels wonderful. The hot glow melts social distinctions and equalizes asymmetry: *they* may have more power, money, and prestige, but *we* are morally superior; they may have the ability to frustrate or terminate our research, but we have the ability to reveal their bad faith and denounce their wrongs. Indignation is seductive, addictive; it's a kind of moral masturbation. As with masturbation, however, the glow is sterile and unproductive.

The problem with anger is that it leads only to blame, not to understanding. Those who practice the ethnography of indignation may be able to expose the misbehavior of the powerful, but exposure, although valuable, cannot help us understand why they behave this way. The hot glow of anger coarsens our perceptions—the perceptions that enable field-workers to do intuitive, insightful, effective research. Lacking empathy and identification, the ethnographer cannot penetrate the subjective reality of the Other. This understanding is as crucial when "studying up" as when "studying down." If we listen to the powerful people we observe only to disqualify what they say, we will be unable to truly hear them, to truly know them as fellow human beings.

This disqualification-in-advance of the people one studies leads to serious misperceptions and misunderstandings. (It also leads to a certain snide or nasty quality to the ethnographer's descriptions and analyses and to an air of righteous superiority, as the researcher routinely discounts the statements and beliefs of those studied.) Thus, when sociologist Eliot Freidson[4] discusses physicians' beliefs about the inevitability of medical mistakes, his very language invalidates these beliefs, presenting them as lies or self-interested rationalizations. Freidson's discussion of mistakes is suffused with the "rhetoric of blame."[5] Sociologist Marcia Millman, who employs a similar rhetoric when examining medical mistakes, also discounts doctors' statements and beliefs about these mistakes.[6] Although the behavior Millman describes in her corrosive book on doctors is truly disturbing, the author's outrage blinds her to significant ambiguities and perplexities in the relationships between doctors and patients.[7]

Observers who are unable (or unwilling) to understand the interrelationships that produce victimization sacrifice the possibility of rectifying such situations. Because the ethnography of indignation depersonalizes those studied, it leads to one-dimensional findings that have power only to generate further indignation rather than social change. To change people's behavior, we must understand *why* they behave as they do. To understand, we must empathize with the people we study, rather than invalidate their reality and humanity. We take this for granted when studying down. But somehow, when many ethnographers study up, the basic precepts go out the window as they substitute the seductive pleasures of the hot glow of anger for the effort to understand.

During thirty-three months of research, I observed appalling conduct by venal, careless, and incompetent surgeons. At the same time, I encountered inspiring behavior by exemplary surgeons, whose clarity, competence, and caring were acknowledged by patients, colleagues, and subordinates. I've attempted in this book to follow the Spinoza epigraph: "not to ridicule, not to deplore, not to denounce, but to understand." In Chapter 6, for example, I present a social drama, wherein an Old-Time Prima Donna takes a shortcut and performs a procedure that ends in the death of his patient. Merely denouncing this man, without exploring his connections to patients and colleagues, and examining changes in the relations between doctors and patients in America (where old-time patients are becoming as extinct as the old-time doctors who cared for them), would negate any possibility of understanding, and consequently coping with, such actions. This understanding is an essential step in initiating significant changes in the behavior of the powerful.

THE WAY OF SAYING

Writing to please has something to be said for it, at least
as against writing to intimidate.

Clifford Geertz
Works and Lives: The Anthropologist as Author

Let us now consider authorial voice. As I explicate my way of
saying, the reader will learn more about my what and why of
saying.

I'll begin with two assertions. Both should be unnecessary, but in today's social science climate, I must belabor the
obvious:[8]

1. My simplicity of style is intentional; it does not stem from
   an inability to negotiate polysyllables, complexity, or jargon.
2. My restriction of citations to those that might advance
   my argument is also intentional; I have read more than I
   have cited.

Strathern notes that "over the last 20 years, certain apparent dichotomies between writer, audience, and subject have
folded in on themselves."[9] The dichotomies fold in when,
for example, Strathern keeps her Melanesian informants in
mind as she describes Melanesian marriage ceremonies,[10] or
when Spencer suggests that the best practical way to vali-
date competing interpretations is to include "subjects" in the
interpretive communities to which anthropological texts are
addressed.[11] The "folding in" in this book is deliberate; my
audience includes my "subjects" and *their* "subjects"; I have
written this book for surgeons, patients, other medical specialists—*and* for social scientists.

The book, then, addresses an intelligent reader who is not
necessarily conversant with social science theory nor willing
to cope with social-science jargon. I've tried to communicate to

this audience my experience of the surgeons I studied and my interpretation of their experience. I have utilized every means I could think of to communicate this experiential knowledge. I've employed narrative when effective,[12] theory when it would advance my argument, quotations from surgeons, exposition, analysis. Rather than stemming from a full-fledged "discursive strategy," the book was put together by a process of *bricolage*.

The simplicity of my style stems not only from the breadth of my audience; simplicity and clarity are also my preference. It's not that I resent scholarship or erudition. It's just that I find a certain kind of academic, trendy, razzle-dazzle glitter unappealing; in such writing, the scholarship draws attention to the *scholar* rather than the subject. It all seems designed to say, "Look at me; look how smart I am!" rather than "Look at my subject of study; think about my ideas." Such writing is fundamentally unserious. (I think of this as being a masculine display, rather like a peacock unfolding his tail, but I could be wrong.)

I find equally unappealing another academic presentation of self: a kind of heavy-handed literalness, an overly boring, Germanic, passive-voiced, verb-absent style, incorporating a hit-the-reader-over-the-head citation of everyone who ever sneezed in the key of D major, if that's the key one is writing in. Such writing is *too* serious. (I think of this as the "good-little-graduate-student-girl" mode, but then, again, I could be wrong.) [13]

In the end, I try to write what I like to read: serious, unostentatious writing, where the scholarly scaffolding is employed to illuminate the subject of study rather than the competencies of the author, where the theorizing flows directly from the data rather than the data being crammed into preexisting theory, and where abstractions and scholarly speculation are leavened by personal sentiment and narrative.[14]

Although I trust that medical anthropologists and sociologists will find my material interesting and useful, they are not my primary audience. If these scholars conclude, "She's not doing medical anthropology" (or sociology), they'll be right. I'm not, really. The book is closer to a classic ethnography— of a savage, exotic, secluded tribe. (That the tribe lives among us makes it all the more interesting—especially since we encounter surgeons at work primarily when we are naked, horizontal, and unconscious.)

A number of contemporary ethnographic critics endorse textual simplicity when it issues from a scholar safely ensconced in the past. As a historic communication, simplicity can be characterized, in somewhat elegiac tones, as "transparency." [15] (Here we encounter the professorial version of the pastoral, situating earlier field-workers in a kind of epistemological Eden, where they lack the fatal self-consciousness that burdens our postmodern reflections.) The same critics, however, tend to ignore or denigrate contemporary ethnographies that lack the scholarly scaffolding, ritual invocations of European theorists, analytic acrobatics, and social-science locutions that mark the writer as "one of us." Such work, they assume, must be a product of ignorance, or more reprehensible still, a desire to popularize, to exchange one's intellectual birthright for money, media recognition, and the admiration of those unwilling or unable to penetrate the thickets of contemporary social-science discourse. [16] Such critics do not comprise a significant portion of my intended audience.

A REFLEXIVE TURN

Positivist social science has not considered the full description of experience as its task, leaving it instead to art and literature. In contrast, anthropology has long had a rhetoric that encompasses the representation of its subjects' experience, even though its guiding concepts and writing conventions have not facilitated the substantive achievements of this rhetoric. Ethnographies of experience are now trying to make full use of the knowledge that the anthropologist achieves from fieldwork, which is much richer and more diverse than what he has been able to distill into conventional analytic monographs.

> George E. Marcus and Michael M. J. Fischer
> *Anthropology as Cultural Critique:*
> *An Experimental Moment in the Human Sciences*

The problem, to rephrase it in as prosaic terms as I can manage, is to represent the research process in the research product; to write ethnography in such a way as to bring one's interpretations of some society, culture, way of life, or whatever and one's encounters with some of its members, carriers, representatives, or whomever into an intelligible relationship. Or . . . how to get an I-witnessing author into a they-picturing story.

> Clifford Geertz
> *Works and Lives: The Anthropologist as Author*

I have made no attempt in this book to transform myself into a detached, "objective" observer in order to create typologies, construct theories, and discover the Platonic reality underlying the booming, buzzing confusion of the field. That I cast myself as an actor in the ethnographic situation will not surprise anthropologists familiar with recent developments in the discipline.[17] Sociologists, on the other hand, may be offended by this approach and by my unapologetic nonpositivism. Those who believe that the job of social science is, in the words of a reviewer who found this manuscript exasperating, "to create typologies and theories which are logical and substantially supported by data" will also agree with that reviewer in finding my work closer to a personal memoir than a social scientific study.[18]

Reflexivity is probably an acquired taste—and one that not everyone acquires. I find the presence of the ethnographic observer *more,* not *less,* scientific: pretending one is invisible or transparent has a certain resemblance to Winnie the Pooh's holding a balloon and hoping that he looks like a cloud rather than a bear with a balloon, seeking honey. (This is not to advocate the solipsistic hall-of-mirrors approach, where the ethnographer becomes so enamored of her own reflection that the people studied are eclipsed by the author's narcissistic self-involvement.)

The ethnographer in this book is an embodied voice, not the disembodied authority of "social science"; she is studying other embodied human beings, not an abstract and orderly "social structure." That I am who I am, not another fieldworker, with my unique personal history, social position, intellectual and emotional biases, is central to this work. It is the confrontation of my person with the unique persons I encountered in the field that produced this particular research product. To understand fully the book and the surgeons I studied, the reader should know who I am, where I was, what I was doing in the field, and what I thought as particular events unfolded.

THE I-WITNESSING AUTHOR

The ethnographer, as a positioned subject, grasps certain human phenomena better than others. He or she occupies a position or structural location and observes with a particular angle of vision. . . . The notion of position also refers to how life experiences both enable and inhibit particular kinds of insight.

Renato Rosaldo
Culture and Truth: The Remaking of Social Analysis

When anthropologists include themselves as characters
in ethnographic texts instead of posing as objective controlling narrators, they expose their biases.

> Frances Mascia-Lees, Patricia Sharpe,
> and Colleen Ballerino Cohen
> "The Postmodernist Turn in Anthropology"

My attitude toward the surgeons I studied is overdetermined.[19]
Although indignation is not temperamentally congenial to
me, another factor affected my perspective: while conducting
fieldwork, I was married to a doctor. (My former husband is
an internist, not a surgeon.)

Renato Rosaldo quotes political theorist Michael Walzer in
saying that the ideal social position for a critic is to be mean-
ingfully connected with the group under critique—not necessarily at the center of things, but neither a complete stranger
nor a spectator.[20] By this criterion, my position for studying
surgeons was exemplary.

Millman, on the other hand, when discussing fieldwork
among doctors, cautions that the ethnographer must not forget that observer and observed "dwell on opposite sides of the
group fence," the ethnographer being "outside," the doctors
"inside."[21] My experience contravened her proscriptions. During fieldwork, I was to some extent on the doctors' side of the
fence: I understood their approach, their point of view, many
of their problems. In certain ways—not all, by any means—
I was an insider, although many of the surgeons I hoped to
study perceived me as an annoying, importunate, and potentially dangerous outsider. This rendered me more sympathetic
to their concerns, more disposed to believe their assertions (at
first hearing, at least), and probably more accepted by the surgeons, as a doctor's wife and social equal. (Whether or not the
surgeons perceived me as a social equal, I perceived myself as
such, which made me more relaxed when they talked down
to me—which many surgeons tend to do to nonsurgeons.)

This book was written when, after thirty years of marriage, I was no longer a doctor's wife. I now perceive my new status as an outsider, not only when talking to doctors but also when interacting with doctors' secretaries and nurses. This gives me a curious double vision, a Picasso-like view of the world of doctors that is shared to some extent by all ethnographers, who perceive reality from both the inside and the outside, through the eyes of those studied and the eyes of the outside world.

I believe my insider/outsider position was an advantage. My "structural location," as Rosaldo would term it, enabled certain insights. During the process of research, I realized how much I knew that I did not know I knew about the lives and attitudes of doctors. I attempted to use this knowledge in this book and to be as clear as possible about where it came from. Naturally, as Rosaldo would also point out, my structural location and life experiences also *inhibited* other insights.

Trying to appeal to as wide an audience as I have runs a risk. Addressing doctors and patients, laypersons and social scientists, can mean that the book will satisfy few. Although I have the traditional ethnographer's affection for her "tribe," I've tried not to take sides, which may anger both surgeons, who want an apologia, and critics, who seek an attack. In the end, all I can say is that I've tried to produce an honest, insightful, knowledgeable, and interesting ethnography of surgeons at work. Observing people, reflecting on my observations, and fitting those observations into larger conceptions of human beings, their desires, activities, and possibilities are ideal activities for a born voyeur like me. This book is an attempt to communicate my vision to a larger audience.

ACKNOWLEDGMENTS

I am grateful to the surgeons who, some willingly, some reluctantly, permitted me to observe their operations, their office hours, their "corridor consultations," who endured my questions and allowed me to tag along as they raced through corridors and up and down back stairs, making rounds, reading X rays, ordering tests, scheduling procedures. My thanks also to the house officers who explained technical details as though I were a particularly ignorant medical student for whose education they held some responsibility. In retrospect, I'm even grateful to those surgeons who did their best—and their best was very good—to frustrate my research. Some flatly refused to allow me to follow and observe them; others assented and then managed time and again to evade me in the maze-like hospital corridors; and one man would loudly announce as I came into view (sometimes holding his nose with one hand and making a flushing gesture with the other), "Here she is again (groan); watch out, she's writing down everything we say!" I learned a lot from them too.

My greatest debt is to the first chief of surgery, who let me in to do fieldwork despite the warnings of colleagues and—I suspect—his own misgivings. That he did so was a testimony to his devotion to his profession, which, overriding fears about risks, fostered the hope that my research might benefit surgeons and surgery.

My thanks to H. Russell Bernard, for suggesting I write the review article that gave me the idea for the study and for encouragement during the writing of this book. My thanks also to Arthur Kleinman, Jonathan Benthal, and Sybil Wolfram, for publishing some rather unconventional anthropological essays based on my material.

The following physicians read all or part of the book: Herbert Yousem, Adrienne Krausz, Elsie Meyer, Roy Mendelsohn, Donald Becker. I am grateful for their comments and advice. Renate and James Fernandez reviewed the manuscript and went far beyond the minimal responsibilities of reviewers in their meticulous, knowledgeable, helpful recommendations for improving it. William F. May suggested references, discussed ethical concepts, and reviewed the chapter on misbehavior, making valuable theoretical and elegant editorial comments. I am grateful to Judith McCulloh for her kindness and enthusiasm and for an editorial suggestion that, suddenly and simply, made the final chapter "work."

My thanks to the National Endowment for the Humanities, which funded the research (Grant #RH2051484).

Murray Wax discussed interpretations, theories, and events, and read and commented on successive versions of each chapter. His intellectual integrity, editorial acumen, and emotional support enabled me to produce this very individual, idiosyncratic book, rather than a more conventional effort.

EXPECTED
MIRACLES

INTRODUCTION

The Surgical "Miracle"

*I*N *A BOOK* about surgeons, it is appropriate to begin with an operation. I shall be prodigal and begin with two.

WORKING A MIRACLE

"Another miracle!" said Raoul, the chief resident, leaving the operating room, where he and an attending surgeon had just performed an emergency operation on Mr. Heinz Neumann, age sixty-nine, who had arrived at the emergency room some hours earlier, in pain, with an enormously distended abdomen. He had an obstructed colon, which might rupture and spread feces and infection throughout the abdomen. The operation had been messy. The colon had bled copiously, and a vast quantity of loose, noxious-smelling fecal material had poured from the bowel, covering towels and white gauze pads, filling the pan a nurse held to catch it. This was Raoul's second emergency operation that afternoon and his third emergency procedure: he had also helped successfully resuscitate a patient who had "coded" in the recovery room after an operation. Mentioning miracles, Raoul's tone was ironic and self-distancing, but, responding to a comment about his busy day, the young surgeon said fervently: "I love it!"

How could he not? Mr. Neumann, pale, almost blue-faced, near death, with an immensely distended abdomen, had been transformed into a rosy-cheeked man with normal-looking contours under his sheet, who smiled at us several days later from his bed in the intensive care unit. The patient's metamorphosis, from near-death to life, was—miraculous.

SEEKING A MIRACLE

"Four of the six patients we're doing today are crazy," said Dr. Villar. "We don't put a psychiatric diagnosis on their chart; that labels them. We say that the patient suffers from Munchausen's syndrome, and other doctors know what we mean. Sometimes we put it in Latin!" (A patient with Munchausen's syndrome invents or induces symptoms, going from hospital to hospital to receive treatment and operations.) "These patients are 'punted' from medicine to surgery," he said. "The internists don't know what to do with them and hope we can figure something out. Of course, we'd like to send them back to the medical doctors if we could; we call it 'turfing' the patient." He said that Mrs. Morelli complains of pains all over her abdomen, remarking: "She's going to look like a checkerboard by the time we're finished. What I'm really practicing is psychiatric surgery," he complained.

Before she was anesthetized, Villar asked the patient to point to all the places on her abdomen that hurt, marking each with a ballpoint pen. Although he had talked as if nothing he could do would really help the patient, while operating, Villar sounded hopeful that he would find something that would make her better. As they removed small pieces of tissue from each of the eight locations Mrs. Morelli had pointed to, Villar and the intern agreed that they looked a little unusual; perhaps there was something wrong that the procedure would help. Since the patient had also complained that the scar from a previous operation hurt, they also removed that.

The next day, Yehuda, a fourth year surgical resident, went over Mrs. Morelli's chart with me. The pathology report said that the surgeons had removed "adipose tissue." "That's just fat!" said Yehuda. He went through the chart, commenting on what he found: "She's had ten operations and she's only thirty-six—that's a bad sign. Three of them are laminectomies [operations on the spine]; that's unheard of! Then, she's allergic to penicillin. She's a nut case!" he exploded. "She has all the signs! Crazy patients often have lots of allergies. And all those operations! And look, she's getting Valium, and another drug I think is a tranquilizer, as well." "What would you do with a patient like that?" I inquired.

"I'd listen to her and be nice to her and try to get her to trust me," he said. "Then I'd try to convince her *not* to get operated on. And if I couldn't convince her, I'd turf her to [the nearby city], to a university hospital, and let them figure out what to do." "Why does Villar operate, then?" I asked. "He loves to operate," explained the resident, "and he likes to take cases no one else will touch."

Mr. Neumann's operation was termed a "miracle" by the chief resident. Although he used an ironic tone, he may well have found the patient's transformation miraculous. Let us briefly consider the characteristics of miracles, to learn why they are so frequently attributed to surgeons.

A miracle is *rapid*. It does not unfold; it occurs. A cure that takes months may be remarkable and gratitude-inducing, but it is not miraculous. Medical care has been discussed as a process extending through time. Surgery, on the other hand, is based upon a finite event: the operation. Although processes such as preoperative and postoperative care affect outcome, the central act in surgery occurs in a measurable, sharply delimited period of time.

A miracle is *spectacular*. Consisting of a reversal or transformation, it propels the beneficiary from a disvalued to a valued state: sickness to health, death to life, water to wine.

It is *definitive*. The beneficiary was sick, is well; disease was excised; the patient is cured. The surgical miracle is irreversible; the patient's body will never be the same.

A miracle is *attributable*. Everyone knows who was responsible.

It is *performed by someone with extraordinary powers*. Specialized knowledge and training, access to marvelous substances, or a relation to mystical or supernatural forces can be cited to explain these powers.

A miracle is *unpredictable and mysterious*. Although it may be involved with rationality, in some ways it transcends rational, known, natural forces; it inspires hope, fear, and wonder.

Some surgical miracles are more marvelous than others. A kind of gambler's calculus determines the dimensions of the miracle,[1] tallying the chance of a favorable outcome and what is being wagered. Most surgical miracles are relatively routine, with a high probability of success and comparatively little risked in case of failure. For patients, naturally, few procedures are routine; the odds are better known by surgeons than patients, and fear and discomfort magnify subjective risk. Moreover, statistical odds cannot predict the outcome of today's encounter between this particular patient and this surgeon in this operating room. An element of uncertainty, of mystery, abides. As the probability of success decreases and that which is risked becomes more perilous—or "consequential"[2]—the more extraordinary the miracle. Operations that triumph over desperate odds and life-threatening risks delight surgeons, who replay the details to colleagues and flaunt their victories at surgical "grand rounds."[3] These are the spectacular miracles patients pray for and the media celebrate.

Seeking such transformations, patients and their families journey to the secular shrines where they are reputed to occur. When a miracle is achieved, the patient never forgets the person who performed it. Surgeons are frequently approached by someone who announces with emotion: "You saved my life!" (Often, the details must be recapitulated before the surgeon remembers the person or procedure.) Some will confide to the surgeon's companion: "I love him!"

The second operation, on Mrs. Morelli, catered to the patient's desire for a miracle. Those who suffer from symptoms that no treatment can relieve do not get malicious pleasure from fooling their doctors. They are in pain; they seek relief. The relief they seek is rapid, spectacular, transformative—in short, miraculous. Patients like Mrs. Morelli pose a terrible problem for physicians. Too "modern" for faith healing, unwilling to accept a psychiatric label for their disorder, in too much pain to live with their symptoms, they haunt doctors' offices, complaining, cajoling, demanding. A permanent reminder of the doctor's impotence in the face of their suffering, such patients drive their physicians wild. They wear out doctors, traveling from one to the next, one hospital to the next, seeking the panacea that will relieve their pain. Whether Mrs. Morelli suffered from Munchausen's syndrome (inducing symptoms that baffled her doctors) or hypochondriasis (fearing disease for which her doctors could find no evidence) or hysteria (displaying symptoms caused by psychic conflict), she aspired to a cure beyond the reach of surgery. Some surgeons, perhaps more arrogant, perhaps less honest, than others, try to treat patients like her, hoping against hope that their procedures will help relieve their pain. Dr. Villar's operation was equivalent to a laying on of hands. Rather than helping her, his "psychiatric surgery" harmed the patient by playing into her fantasy of a miraculous cure. This can surely be termed misbehavior. Faith may be an important, even necessary, ingredient for surgical miracles, but only when the patient suffers from a surgical disorder.

✳

Two operations. Two ways of treating patients. Miraculous surgery, which saves lives; magical surgery, which reaches for impossible miracles. At this point, we could contrast the surgeon patients seek, the one who performs miracles, with the surgeon critics deplore, the one who performs unnecessary operations. Such a scheme is seductive but overly simplistic. The same faith in the near-magical powers of the surgeon animates Dr. Villar and Mrs. Morelli. Charismatic healers, endowed with the gift of grace, must believe in their powers in order to exercise them, and many surgeons possess such a belief in their remarkable powers. This gives them the confidence to cut into human flesh, the daring to move swiftly and surely in the hidden recesses of the body, the tenacity to keep trying when the odds are against them. The line between surgical virtues and vices—between surgeons' confidence and their hubris, their courage and their recklessness—may be, on occasion, uncomfortably narrow.

I am not defending the operation on Mrs. Morelli, which was unwarranted. But, neither am I intimating, as do some critics, that all surgeons are knife-happy butchers who should and must be curbed. What I am suggesting is that a certain ambiguity exists about the performance and motives of surgeons such as Villar. Rather than characterizing such men, with their macho, martial appetite for challenge, as unmitigated villains or charlatans, we would do better to realize that many of the qualities we seek in our surgeons have their shadow side. It is too easy (for patients, surely) to glorify, to perceive the surgeons who save their lives as somehow larger than life. It is just as easy (for social scientists, surely) to debunk, to portray surgeons as clowns, whose actions are motivated solely by venality, vanity, or foolhardiness. Distinguishing dualities is simple: black or white, good or evil. Ambiguities are more difficult for patients and social scientists to grasp.

Naturally, the term "miracle" is a metaphor. And, "the essence of metaphors is understanding and experiencing one thing in terms of another." [4] In this book, I use this focal metaphor of the miracle to illuminate the behavior, interactions, and misunderstandings of surgeons and patients.

The metaphor of the miracle has religious antecedents, as do other metaphors I use. In this book, I explore the mysterious, transcendent dimension of the surgeon's art, considering the ritual aspects of surgery and the priestly role of the surgeon; characterize surgeons' remarks about their colleagues as a kind of medieval morality play; explore deadly surgical sins; and cite Dostoyevski's haunting parable of the Grand Inquisitor to reflect on the relation between the charismatic powers of the surgeon and patients' longing for miracle, mystery, and authority. These metaphors highlight a rarely discussed aspect of surgeons' relation to their work. Cutting into the human body is a terrifying undertaking, and the ritual of surgery, "at once murderous, painful, healing, and full of love,"[5] evokes an ineffable sense of mystery and awe in its practitioners.

My argument in this book is relatively simple and—when compared to burning exposées and denunciations—unsensational: that everything has a price, and miracles are no exception. We get nothing for nothing. In the following chapters, I show how the miraculous qualities of successful operations influence the attitudes, expectations, and behavior of the surgeons who perform them; the "paranoia" of those who fail to produce them; the expectations of the patients who submit to them; and the rage of those for whom they are not produced. I examine the charismatic authority of surgeons, its instability, and its price, and the price of substituting bureaucratic structures for that charisma. The "disenchantment of the world" has a cost for surgeons, whose commitment and joy are eroded, and for patients, whose healing faith and trust are diminished.

This book demonstrates that operations, such as the procedures undergone by Mr. Neumann and Mrs. Morelli, do not occur in a vacuum; they take place among a "fellowship" or community of surgeons who practice at the same hospital, supervised by a chief of surgery, responsible for training young surgeons and monitoring the work of senior men. The community of surgeons is embedded in a larger community, whose inhabitants discuss their doctors with one another and seek to impose their own beliefs and demands upon them. The book examines the community of surgeons to illustrate how they influence, criticize, and protect one another. We go behind the scenes in the hospital to settings where patients never penetrate; overhear conversations about patients, families, colleagues; encounter pointed remarks masquerading as jokes about colleagues whose behavior is sanctioned; observe operations, patient rounds, and office hours; and explore the values, attitudes, behavior, and misbehavior of the surgeons we observe.

This is not an exposée, a "hate surgeons" book. Nor is it a paean to the noble, misunderstood, and unfairly maligned surgeon. I describe what I observed during thirty-three months of anthropological research among surgeons, analyze the meanings of these observations, and indicate how the benefits associated with modern surgery and the surgeons who perform its miracles have their inevitable costs, as well as how attempts to reduce those costs may also have their own unanticipated price.

1

THE ART, CRAFT, AND SCIENCE OF MIRACLES

> The wounded surgeon plies the steel
> That questions the distempered part;
> Beneath the bleeding hands we feel
> The sharp compassion of the healer's art
> Resolving the enigma of the fever chart.
>
> T. S. Eliot
> "East Coker"

> Nor is practical wisdom concerned with universals only
> —it must also recognize the particulars; for it is practical,
> and practice is concerned with particulars.
>
> Aristotle
> *Nicomachean Ethics*

TO SPEAK of surgery as "miraculous" is both metaphorical and wishful. Successful surgery does, in truth, display some of the characteristics of miracles. But, unlike miracles, surgery is based upon knowledge, training, and technology; it is fathomable and explicable; and its principles and techniques can be imparted to others.

Surgery is an art, a craft, and a science, which explains why surgeons rarely mention miracles, except "jokingly."[1] Surgeons know they cannot brandish a scalpel, utter an in-

9

cantation, and become a conduit for supernatural forces. The surgeon must *make* the miracle happen.

It is the more rational, perceptible aspects of surgery that determine the characteristics of a good surgeon. And yet, even here, some mystery lingers; some gifts emerge that resist testing, quantification, verification. Even here, we find individuals with powers that may be perceived by colleagues as a kind of grace or charisma.

This chapter examines the attributes surgeons evaluate, admire, and emulate in colleagues. It then indicates how few of these can be perceived by patients and suggests that these areas of incomprehension may reinforce patients' belief in and hope for miracles.

THE GOOD SURGEON: COLLEAGUES' EVALUATIONS

Let us begin with four descriptions of the same man:[2]

> He's extremely compassionate, extremely competent, not condescending in the least—and he *cares*, that's very important.

> He has judgment, knowledge, character and skill.

> He has good academics, good background, looks the role, has good technical ability, takes care of the folks.

> He's a gentleman, he does not raise his voice, he's considerate to the patient and gives excellent care. He's there when necessary, makes good judgments when surgery should be done and not done. Of course, I wouldn't mind having a car [Ferrari] like his as well!

Some of these attributions are not surprising. Others are, perhaps, unexpected. Let us examine the characteristics colleagues admire and emulate, beginning with the most basic requirement for a good surgeon.

Good Hands

Fundamental to a good surgeon is technical proficiency, or "good hands." Lacking technical skill, a surgeon may be a good *doctor*, but never a good surgeon. A house officer told me that a senior surgeon, whose personal and professional behavior he described as "sleazy," had very good hands. "He's an elegant surgeon," he said. When one observes a surgeon with "good hands" operate, everything looks easy, almost inevitable; the performance has a kind of rhythm, speed, and flow. Even emergencies, such as an unexpected hemorrhage, appear to be under control. Surgeons describe such colleagues admiringly, as a "superb technician," a "brilliant technical surgeon," a "good operator." Of a man characterized as "the absolute essence of the ideal general surgeon," a young surgeon said: "He just had the most incredibly gifted hands. You could compare him to Michelangelo. That's how much of a pleasure it was to operate with him and watch him."

A technically gifted practitioner, then, may be perceived as transforming the craft of surgery into an art; such artistry can be admired and emulated, but never fully explained. During an operation, a surgeon who taught at a medical school remarked that his opinion had changed about technique. He used to think there was nothing in it when people ascribed successes to someone's technique, but he's since learned that: "some guys can do things no one else can get away with, and it always turns out well. While other people have to be twice as careful." As he spoke, this right-handed surgeon tied an elegant "one-handed surgeon's knot" with his left hand. The one-handed surgeon's knot, where one hand holds a length of thread taut while the fingers of the other hand deftly contrive square knots with a second length of thread, is a bravura display of technical facility. It's performed quietly. If one does not recognize the maneuver one may miss it—as I did, during my first year and a half of watching operations. I've observed only two surgeons do a one-handed knot with their weaker hand; another tied one while looking away from his hands and talking to a colleague. A house officer told how he had once joked about a senior surgeon's fingers being too thick for the one-handed knot. The man became very upset, stopped the operation, made everyone wait, and slowly tied a one-handed knot. Not every surgeon performs the one-handed knot, and not every surgeon approves of it—but every senior surgeon and surgical house officer understands its meaning: the knot both demonstrates and signifies technical facility. "When I was a house officer," said one man, while cutting with his left hand and tying one-handed knots with his right, "you weren't supposed to do these. That's silly!" he added. A chief of surgery, on the other hand, told me that he doesn't like "tricks" and that he tells his house officers who try things such as the one-handed knot: "You're in danger because you have good hands. Forget that, it's *judgment* [that counts]!"

Superb technique wins the admiration of house staff and colleagues, but technical facility untempered by knowledge and judgment can be dangerous, seducing surgeons into procedures that more prudent colleagues avoid. Harshly echoing an opinion prevalent in his hospital, about a surgeon with superb technical facility and a high record of complications, an intern said: "He's got great hands—too bad he's dead from the neck up!" And, "cut here" was the way a chief characterized the surgeon with good hands who relies upon the referring physician to tell him what is wrong with the patient and what to do about it.

Knowledge

To be more than a hired knife, a surgeon must have knowledge—of disorders, diseases, procedures, and treatments. I've heard surgeons contrast two kinds of knowledge: *personal, experiential* knowledge and *scientific* knowledge.[3] The contrast may, at times, reflect a tension between nonacademic practitioners of surgery and "full-time" academic surgeons, who divide their time between teaching, research, and performing surgery.

Practicing surgeons frequently discuss cases in terms of personal experience: "I've seen this before, the best way to deal with it is . . ."; "I've got a gut feeling this is a . . ."; "In twenty years, I've only seen one of these!" Experiential knowledge includes not only what can go wrong with the human body, but also the various ways in which the body may be constructed. When I began to observe operations, I was surprised to learn that anatomy is not geography, that no single road map can depict the byways of the human body. During operations I'd hear phrases such as "Whaddya know, he's got three!" or, "Wow, this one turns to the *left!*"

Let me note that laypersons and medical critics (and those who set medical reimbursements) are apparently unaware that in surgery, as in all of medicine, *there are no interchangeable parts.* Disorders differ, physiological reactions differ, even anatomy differs from patient to patient. In similar fashion, surgeons differ; *one surgeon is not interchangeable with another.* This is an elementary observation; yet many patients and critics, while conceding their own psychic and social uniqueness, seem to ignore their physiological and anatomical uniqueness—as well as the personal and technical uniqueness of each doctor who treats them.

Surgeons' experiential knowledge covers variation in anatomy, disorders, and procedures. The longer a surgeon has been in practice, the more variation he is likely to have encountered. "I've been doing this for thirty years," an older surgeon habitually proclaimed to dissenting colleagues. Such an argument has a certain validity.

In university hospitals, the "full-time" surgeons, who teach medical students and house officers, stress scientific knowledge. When house officers at these elite institutions present cases to colleagues and seniors, they are expected to be familiar with the most recent research findings and to cite the probable outcomes of various treatments and procedures. During case discussions, senior surgeons question residents, making it clear by their questions and their responses to the questions of colleagues just what sort of knowledge the residents are expected to master.[4]

On occasion, I have heard "town" and "gown" express mutual distrust of each other's knowledge bases. Practitioners have intimated that although academic surgeons may have book knowledge, they lack sufficient on-the-ground experience about what can and does occur when a patient is open before one on the operating table; while academics subtly (or not so subtly) have denigrated the practitioners' ignorance of the latest literature, statistics, techniques, and procedures. The practitioners' accusation might roughly be summed up as, "He knows a lot, but can't *do* much"; the academics' taunt is, "He does a lot, but doesn't *know* much."

Naturally, both kinds of knowledge are essential for the surgeon who operates, as opposed to one who confines himself to teaching or research. Academic surgeons do, in fact, exhibit experiential knowledge—although it is perhaps not as broad as that of their practitioner colleagues; and practitioners do exhibit book learning—although it is perhaps not as profound as that of their academic colleagues. Some practitioners (not all, by any means) may rely primarily upon the books and journals they read as medical students and house officers.

Whether experiential or academic, however, medical knowledge is *general*. The surgeon may have seen six, eight, or a hundred cases resembling this one in some respects; he may know that a recent study indicates that a certain percentage of people with a particular disorder, manifested by certain symptoms, treated in a certain fashion, will exhibit a particular outcome. Deciding what *this specific case* might be, however, whether this specific patient's symptoms add up to this specific disease (which involves deciding which similarities to notice and which to ignore), and then deciding how to handle this particular case, requires clinical skills, or judgment.

Judgment

Clinical judgment involves application of the surgeon's general knowledge to the specific case at hand. The young surgeon who described the "absolute essence of the ideal general surgeon" admired not only the man's gifted hands but also his formidable clinical skills: "His clinical judgment was impeccable, the man was never wrong! His clinical acumen was totally beyond belief, it was like a real sixth sense." Even more important than knowing how to cut, one surgeon told me, is knowing when to operate, when to stop cutting, and how to take care of what you did.

Diagnosing what is wrong with a patient requires clinical judgment. So, then, does deciding what to do, including a decision to do nothing; a surgeon, I was told, can be judged by the cases he refuses as well as how skillfully he handles those he accepts. Refusing to operate on a patient one cannot help is not easy for surgeons, who tend to be activists. They are tempted to do something, *anything*. The following interchanges took place at a "mortality and morbidity" (M and M) conference, where cases that have resulted in death or complications are discussed:

> A resident presented the case of an eighty-four-year-old man, who had arrived in the emergency room with a large, black, foul-smelling length of gangrenous bowel. This was removed, but the patient died. When the decision to operate was questioned, the house officer and the chief of surgery both agreed that the patient had not been viable from the first. The house officer, however, claimed that it would have been difficult to present a decision *not* to operate to the patient's family, and the usually critical chief did not contradict his argument.

(A decision to do *nothing* is courageous, "unsurgical," and rare [5]—which may be one reason why so many intensive care units are filled with moribund patients in their eighties and nineties who have had procedures with little potential to slow their impending demise.)

If he chooses to operate, the surgeon must then decide what procedure to perform and how it will be done (e.g., what kind of incision; where the incision will be; what kind of thread; what types of stitches; whether to use staples or thread for various joinings and closings). Timing also involves judgment. Is the sick person well enough to operate on immediately, or should the patient be "tuned up" before risking an operation? Is the patient's condition too grave for hesitation; should the operation be performed "emergently"? Postoperative care also requires clinical skills. What kind of antibiotic(s) should be administered to minimize infection, and for how long? If complications arise, such as infection, pneumonia, abscess, and—so dreaded by surgeons they rarely talk about it—"wound dehiscence" [6]—how shall these be treated?

Clinical judgment is difficult, perhaps impossible, for a layperson to observe. It utilizes (as the young surgeon said of the admired senior) a kind of sixth sense. Clinical judgment deals with process,[7] not event; the passage of time is an essential element in the preoperative and postoperative decisions the surgeon must make. Judgment involves the *art* of medicine. "In the world of medicine," reports Bosk, "clinical acumen is a charismatic possession, a gift of grace; its exact nature is a mystery." [8] Opinion differs on how much of this sixth sense can be taught. "I could teach a gorilla to operate in six months," many surgeons say, "but not *when*."

Temperament

A person with the wrong temperament will hesitate in emergencies, have difficulty making decisions, and spend so much time agonizing over what to do that he operates too slowly (see Chapter 2). Lord Hamlet, whose flaw was "thinking too precisely on the event," would have made an abysmal surgeon; it is the martial and decisive Fortinbras, who goes to war "to gain a little patch of ground that hath in it no profit but the name," who exhibits the surgical temperament. Rather than discussing the temperament of colleagues and juniors, surgeons focus upon characteristics that, to an outside observer, may seem somewhat tangential.

> "He looks frail," said a chief of surgery dismissively, of a prospective house officer. Although "frail" was not the term that occurred to me, this particular applicant did seem to lack the confident, athletic, swashbuckling air exhibited by more preferred candidates. Despite the chief's doubts, the candidate, who had excellent recommendations, was accepted into the hospital's training program. He proved to be intelligent, conscientious, hard-working, and beloved by patients. "He's fantastic, one of the three best interns in the country," said his chief resident. The chief admitted he was "very good," but he still expressed misgivings, commenting, "I don't know how he's going to be able to direct everything; he's so retiring." In the middle of his second year, this house officer decided to change specialties. "He's very good," said his new chief resident, "but he has a terrible time making decisions. He can do all the preparation, but he hates to make the actual decision. He'll come to me and ask and be very grateful if it's made for him."

"Frail" is a figure of speech, where the part, the young man's physical presentation of self, represents the whole, the surgical temperament. I suspect that the young surgeon who "jokingly" mentioned his colleague's Ferrari, when asked about the characteristics of his ideal surgeon, was using a similar associative mechanism: the Ferrari demonstrates and symbolizes his colleague's surgical panache.

Personal Qualities

A good surgeon must possess certain attributes that are not quite a matter of temperament, although I am not sure how else to characterize them. The ability to concentrate, for example, is critical. "If you lose your attention for a minute, you can miss something," explained a young surgeon. This concentration involves a capacity to shut out all external and internal stimuli and focus exclusively on the operation at hand.[9] I've observed surgeons operate for more than nine hours without taking a break—for food, water, or toilet. When I commented on their iron bladders, one man responded: "Oh, the adrenaline! You're so concentrated on what you're doing, you just don't think of it." One surgeon told me that although normally she goes to the toilet frequently, she never needs to do so when she operates. She can suffer from a headache or diarrhea, but during the operation, the headache or diarrhea disappear.[10] (The ability to transcend ordinary physical limits when engaged in healing is characteristic of shamans and healers, reported a colleague, who has studied healers in Africa and Alaska.)[11]

Let me note that during thirty-three months studying general surgeons I met only seven women above the rank of house officer. "Surgery is the most male of medical specialties and the least friendly to women," declared a woman surgeon.[12] The surgical temperament involves characteristics that are in our culture traditionally attributed to men: arrogance, aggressiveness, courage, and the ability to make split-second decisions in the face of life-threatening risks. (See the following chapter for an analysis of the temperament of surgeons.) Women surgeons, then, face a double bind: if they have the right temperament, their colleagues may perceive them as "pushy" and "nonfeminine"; if they do not, they will be poor surgeons. Each of the seven senior women surgeons I met and observed at work was remarkable—as indeed she had to be to beat the odds.[13] When, in this book, I refer to general surgeons as "he," I am describing the situation I observed.

The surgeon must also possess a kind of obsessive patience, or even compulsivity—the ability to keep going until every persnickety detail is attended to. Such patience involves self-discipline, which might be considered an aspect of character as well as temperament. Although surgical training stresses it, this attribute is not distributed equally among surgeons. Let's observe this obsessiveness in action, as a surgeon removes a suspicious mass from a woman's breast:

Field Notes.[14] Verdi helped get the table ready, putting arm pieces under the patient's arms. He found the vein for Doris Wu [the anesthesiologist] to insert a needle in for anesthesia; and he helped drape her [the patient]. . . . (He even filled out the form nurses usually fill out, saying what the preliminary diagnosis is!) "She had a needle biopsy, and it was bloody fluid [which could not be analyzed by the pathologist]," he explained. "and you gotta be from Missouri." . . . He showed the resident how the mass was in a bad place for a scar; it would show if the patient wore a bathing suit. . . . Instead, he went in from the rim of the nipple. They hit an artery, though, and the incision bled like mad. "What price beauty, see?" he said to the resident. "Hope she has a low-necked dress!" But, he didn't seem upset; he just kept pushing laps [gauze pads] in, and the bleeding gradually stopped. "If it was me, I hope you wouldn't bother with that, I don't *own* a low-necked dress," said Doris Wu. "Yeah, but if it's a benign cyst, it's a terrible thing to have a bad cosmetic effect," replied Verdi. He showed the resident how he was closing with a special stitch he learned from a plastic surgeon twenty years ago that's good for jagged edges, explaining that he did another kind of stitch on the earlier case [this was his second breast biopsy, assisted by the same house officer] because he'll probably end up doing more on that patient's breast. He was careful to insist on a fresh towel under the patient before they put on the surgical bra so it would not get stained with blood. He even helped put her on the stretcher, although it was 1:35, and he had said he was due to operate in [the nearby big city] at 2:00.

When Dr. Verdi helped drape and prepare the patient, he was making absolutely sure that everything would be done correctly, that no detail would be omitted. He took extra time to make an incision at the nipple and to close with a special stitch to make sure the patient would not exhibit a scar when wearing bathing suits or evening dresses. He even took the trouble to make sure that the white cotton bra that the patient was dressed in when the biopsy was completed was not bloodstained. Such obsessiveness is *unnatural*—when one is tired, or rushed, one tends to take things for granted. But, in surgery, *nothing* can be taken for granted; nothing *should* be taken for granted. This is the lesson young doctors must learn.

> Making rounds in the intensive care unit (ICU) of a public hospital, an attending surgeon, followed by house officers and medical students, explained that sometimes the overworked hospital technicians don't bother to carry out scheduled tests; they just mark the tests as completed, with normal results. "I'm really being paranoid here," he said, pointing out that the results from a particular urine analysis were handwritten, while the machine that performed the analysis usually inserted the numbers automatically. Always redo tests that do not show what you think they should show, he advised.

Such painstakingness, such unwillingness to take anything for granted, to trust anyone else's efforts, may be a kind of necessary suspiciousness, contributing to the "paranoia" of surgeons (see Chapter 2).

Concentration and the willingness to take pains are the first qualities to vanish when a surgeon ages, said one man. "It's not the hands, but the attention span that goes," he explained. "If you're on your feet a long time operating, you may get tired and just want to finish as quickly as you can, so you don't take the pains or keep going as long as perhaps you should. You lose that intense concentration you sometimes need to do what you have to do," he declared.

Caring and Character

Some surgeons mentioned caring and character when they described behavior they admired. Before we return to these and speculate about whether a bad person could be a good surgeon, let us consider how many of these attributes can be observed by patients and their families.

LOOKING UPWARD FROM THE TABLE:
A PATIENT'S-EYE VIEW

Technique

In a surgeon's waiting room, a patient described how, when members of her postmastectomy support group compared scars, she *knew* her stitches were the best. (Despite this confidence, her surgeon had the reputation among his colleagues of having below-average technical dexterity.)

Patients frequently observe their scars and attempt to evaluate their stitches. The smaller the scar, the less visible the surface stitches, the more skill patients are likely to attribute to their surgeons.

Surgeons are aware of patients' evaluations, and one boasted to me about the smallness of his incisions. Some use extra-fine thread to give their patients "plastic [surgery] closings." In reality, however, small scars may not always be good for patients. A surgeon should try to get "good exposure," some surgeons told me, with an incision large enough to see what is going on, and to do the most skillful job possible within the body, rather than concentrating on cosmetic results. With insufficient visibility, a surgeon might be "rough on tissue," causing additional postoperative pain. Consequently, the correlation between surgeons' technical ability and the size of patients' scars and visibility of closing stitches, is imperfect. Surgeons with good hands *and* good judgment may be concentrating on matters they believe more important to the welfare of the patient than postoperative aesthetics. General surgeons who *do* concentrate primarily on aesthetics—during operations where the scar is not visible when the patient is clothed—may have technical facility but be considered by their colleagues to be poor (or sleazy) surgeons because they care more about external characteristics that impress patients than about the long-range well-being of these patients.[15]

Because they often focus on surface phenomena, patients' judgments of their surgeons' technical facility cannot be totally reliable.

Knowledge

Too much disparity exists between the knowledge of laypersons and that of even poorly educated and inexperienced surgeons for patients to be able to observe or estimate the knowledge of their surgeons. It is too easy for someone—even an anthropologist, with surface knowledge and imperfect control of the vocabulary—to appear knowledgeable to unknowing and fearful patients and their families.

Judgment

Clinical judgment is even more difficult than knowledge for a patient to observe. After almost three years of observing surgeons, I was still unable to evaluate judgment. I could observe *results*—and I learned that some surgeons' patients almost always did better than others'—but I had to rely upon house officers (and on occasion colleagues) for evaluations of clinical skills.

Temperament

Patients are in no position to observe surgeons' nerve, concentration, or patience while operating. (They may note the surgeon's patience or impatience with their questions and requests. However, surgeons who possess such interpersonal patience do not necessarily exhibit the obsessive patience for details necessary to successfully diagnose, operate, and care for patients.)

Patients can observe one aspect of a surgeon's temperament: his *confidence*. A surgeon's self-confidence and ability to inspire confidence in patients is manifest. One surgeon told me: "You've got to make patients feel that you think their operation isn't all that serious, that you know you can handle the operation, and that they're going to get better fast." Another spoke of inspiring confidence as a kind of seduction, saying: "You've got to seduce the patient, you've got to convince them that you're the best possible surgeon, that you've got everything under control, that they're going to get better fast. You've got to seduce the referring doctor, convince him you're the best possible person to send the case to. You've got to seduce the family and make them feel confidence in you."

Physical appearance can help instill confidence. Of an admired and respected colleague, a young surgeon remarked, "He's handsome, and that doesn't hurt!" Discussing appearance, one man noted that patients frequently meet their surgeon for the first time when they are told that they need an operation. He explained: "The first impression is very important when the physician-patient relationship begins. When they *look* at you, if you haven't shaved, if you're unclean, disheveled—they're very perceptive. Physical accoutrements are very important—how you carry yourself. It has to do with trust. . . . You have to make them sicker before you make them better. That's why trust is so important. . . . Your physical appearance can help inspire trust." A surgeon in his first year of practice would on occasion joke about patients' distrustful remarks about his youthful appearance. "This is a case for the silver fox," he would say, referring to his handsome, silver-maned surgeon-father.

Not surprisingly, patients also judge surgeons by *results*. They observe the results of their own operations, which depend, to a large extent, on their surgeon's technique, knowledge, and judgment. They also frequently know about the results of other operations performed by the surgeon—in other words, his reputation.

Patients may also evaluate surgeons' trustworthiness (an aspect of character). Patients are usually aware when a surgeon is always there for them. They may not always be able to discern untrustworthiness, but they know when their surgeon consistently comes through for them.

Many patients evaluate caring. People have told me their surgeons were wonderful because they really cared about them; others described how terrible their cold, uncaring surgeons were.

Feedback exists between these characteristics. Patients' confidence is enhanced when they believe their surgeon is trustworthy and when they feel he cares. Confidence is also increased when they know he has achieved excellent results in the past; I was told that famous surgeons inspire confidence—even in patients who have never met them before the operation and who may see them for only a few minutes afterwards. Confidence improves results. Said one surgeon: "Confidence in your recovery has a great deal to do with recovery. You can feel lousy, but if you have confidence in getting better, you will get better." Caring, too, may improve results. "The patient," one man explained, "feels more encouraged, rather than feeling like a slab of meat."

Patients, and on occasion surgeons, may perceive something else for which few words exist. Again, we come to an almost magical or mystical aspect of the doctor-patient relationship: a transaction that enables patients to tap inner resources they did not know they possessed. Many surgeons do not like to talk about this—at least, not to an anthropologist outsider. Surgeons present themselves as rational, technical men of science; discussions of nonlinear, nonrational forces seem to make them uncomfortable. This transaction, or force, has been called *healing*. Some surgeons seem to possess the ability to *heal* patients as well as *cure* them.

Among the characteristics that patients can evaluate, then, are a surgeon's confidence, previous results, trustworthiness (to some extent), and (to some extent) the surgeon's caring. On occasion, patients may experience, even if they cannot evaluate, a kind of healing exchange.

These attributes—confidence, trustworthiness, caring—are all nonlinear, nondiscursive, and nonmeasurable. Even information about previous results may have a random, unpredictable quality. Few patients have access to statistical measures of the outcomes of particular surgeons' operations; instead, patients ask friends about the success or failure of *their* operations, rely upon the judgment and advice of their medical doctors, or, if they can afford it, seek the services of a famed specialist or celebrated hospital (whose results, they trust, are as glowing as their reputations). All the attributes patients are able to evaluate, then, are somewhat mysterious, even magical. When these are combined with the terror and profound neediness of a sick person, we may well find the hope for, belief in, and search for a miracle worker. The result, then, of patients' inability to evaluate surgeons' technique, knowledge, and judgment, may be an overvaluation of the mysterious, nonrational elements in the doctor-patient relationship and an inappropriate reaching after miracles.

CARING AND HEALING

Most surgeons care about their patients, explained an internist, but more than one kind of caring exists in medicine. Surgeons may define their task as caring for patients' *bodies*, he said, or they may define it to include caring for patients *as persons*. Quite naturally, patients want to believe their surgeon cares about them as persons; some surgeons do.

Caring is shown in many ways. A patient may not perceive the actions that express the sentiment, but they *sense* the concern.

> One young surgeon held the hand of an eighty-one-year-old woman between both of his, talking to her in a low, loving, soothing tone before she was anesthetized (to have a cancerous breast mass removed). When the sheet covering her slipped and her breast was uncovered, he did something I've never seen before— or since—he quietly covered the breast again.

Caring behavior is taught—as is uncaring behavior—by observation and precept. One surgeon described how the celebrated man who trained him would sit on patient's beds and touch them. Thirty years later, the surgeon still remembered his mentor's maxim: "Just going by the patient's room is making rounds; going in and sitting down is *visiting* the patient."

Many surgeons have told me that caring (*about* as opposed to *for* a patient) can improve surgical results. They offered different explanations for this. Some said caring makes surgeons more painstaking, or compulsive. (In my experience, the most caring surgeons were, indeed, the most painstaking ones.) A young surgeon, who declared that "you can worry a patient well," explained:

> I think caring about a patient means inquiring about them several times a day, seeing them several times a day. I think seeing a patient several times a day because you care about them can pick up the fact that the NG [nasogastric] tube is not draining well, that it needs to be irrigated. And just by accident—you'll have been in there because you care about the patient—you can fix the NG tube and make it work. Or you can get the electrolytes [16] on the patient, which weren't available at the time you were making rounds in the morning. If you come back in the afternoon, the 'lytes [electrolytes] might be available and IV fluids [intravenous

fluids] might [need to] be changed [because of the electrolyte concentrations].

Caring *about* a patient, in this view, improves caring *for* that patient. Another surgeon explained that caring improves surgeons' communication with patients, and therefore improves patient cooperation. When asked by their surgeon, patients will cough, which is painful but helps avoid pneumonia after chest surgery, or walk, which may also be painful but accelerates postoperative recovery. Another surgeon said he did not know why caring improves results, but he knows that it does. He thought there was probably a scientific reason that had not yet been discovered, perhaps endorphins.

Explaining why caring improves surgical results, one man declared, "organ disease is only a small part of the patient's illness." Here, we encounter the distinction between *illness* and *disease,* much discussed in the past decade.[17] In this distinction, illness, or "patients' experience of disorder"[18] is contrasted with disease, or "abnormalities of the structure and function of body organs and systems."[19] Patients suffer from illness; doctors treat disease. A parallel distinction is drawn between *healing* (relieving the burden of illness) and *curing* (intervening and eradicating or ameliorating the disease process). Healing may occur and illness may be alleviated with no alteration of the underlying disease. Alternatively, a disease may be cured, and yet the patient may feel no better.

When I asked an academic surgeon in charge of the teaching program at an elite medical school if he believed that caring made a difference in patients' getting better, he responded: "Absolutely. No doubt about it! I don't see how you can get people well otherwise. It's accidental without that." He said he teaches this to medical students and house officers, shows them how to sit on the bed, touch the patients. He thinks touching is very important. He talks to patients before operating on them and lets them know he cares. "It's very important for them to know that I want to invade more than their physical space," he said. He told a story that illustrates the link between caring and healing:

> The surgeon had gone to see a patient (the father of a friend), who had arrived, very badly injured, at the emergency room of his hospital. Subsequently, the man was operated on by another surgeon. Months later, the patient said to my informant, "You saved my life!" Not remembering what had happened, the surgeon inquired, and the friend's father reminded him. When the surgeon had entered the emergency room, everyone had been rushing around, caring for this gravely injured man. The surgeon had gone to the patient and said, "You're going to be all right! We're in control." [20]

By caring—and something else, related to caring, which is difficult to describe because it is nondiscursive—this surgeon had acted as a *healer*. This process involves the doctor using himself, his own person, to reach out to the person of the patient.[21] The surgeon's assurance and concern convinced the injured man that he would live. This so impressed the patient that he attributed his very life to the exchange between himself and the surgeon.

Although patients and many surgeons believe caring is important, surgeons, unlike patients, know that caring *about* the patient is useless unless the surgeon possesses the technique, knowledge, and clinical judgment to care adequately *for* that patient. Healing may improve surgical results, but it cannot substitute for those results. The surgical act par excellence is *curing*. As noted, unlike specialties such as internal medicine, whose activities are based primarily upon *processes* played out through time (thus accentuating the healing exchange between physician and patient), at the heart of surgery is an *event*, the operation. During this operation, it is cure—the defeat and excision of disease—that is pursued, not healing. The surgeon seeks, and frequently obtains, definitive results. Disease must be managed, temporized with, outwitted, in surgery as well as in other specialties. But the surgeon offers a possibility of rapid and definitive cure.

A surgeon, then, who heals but lacks the skills to effect a cure, is worthless. Said one man: "Everything boils down to the time of surgery—what did you do during surgery. The rest is window dressing." Caring surgeons without technique, knowledge, and judgment are despised by peers. Such men are perceived as frauds by colleagues—and indeed they are. Such a surgeon is playing on the desire for miracles, without possessing the surgical attributes that *make miracles happen.*

Caring may assume disproportionate emphasis for patients, who are unable to observe and evaluate the art, craft, and science of surgery. It is conceivable that highly educated patients —and critics of medicine—place an even greater stress upon caring than others. Skilled interpersonal exchanges are valued in their milieux, and a surgeon who refuses to converse with them, explain to them, recognize *their* persons, accomplishments, needs, and beliefs may be particularly hurtful.

Surgeons know that laypersons do not understand. I suspect this is why some surgeons, whom I've observed engage in extremely caring behavior, verbally disparage it. When asked whether caring about a patient made that patient better faster, a chief of surgery said dismissively, "Sounds like something that would come out of a nursing study" (a high insult from a rank-conscious surgeon). Some surgeons contrast caring with technique, as though the two were mutually exclusive. Said one, "I'd rather be operated on by a bastard with great technical facility than by a caring nonfacile surgeon."

We might schematicize the relationship between the attributes of a good surgeon by placing them in levels, or layers, each necessary for the one above it. Hands are the fundamental basis: a good surgeon *must* have technical facility. Technique is necessary, but not sufficient; a gorilla can (theoretically) be taught to operate; but a good surgeon must also have knowledge. Medical knowledge is general, however, effective only if the surgeon is able to apply it to specific patients; a good surgeon must possess judgment, or clinical skills. All these characteristics are necessary, even sufficient to being a good surgeon, perhaps even a very good surgeon—if the person is temperamentally suited to the specialty.

If the surgeon has the foundation, hands, knowledge, and clinical judgment, then, *and only then,* can caring about the patient as a person improve results. Without these basic characteristics of a good surgeon, the top layer, caring, is merely "window dressing."

Does this mean that the surgeon is merely a glorified technician?

It means that the surgeon *must* be a glorified technician—and may choose without dishonor to be no more. The dazzling and dramatic technician, who jousts with death and wins, is the surgical hero. "You couldn't have a good surgeon who didn't believe in the concept of the hero," said a chief of surgery. "Every surgical house officer worth his salt would like to be a hero."

The hero may exhibit extraordinary gifts for curing disease, yet possess little aptitude for healing illness. He relegates the latter task, which he perceives as "hand-holding," to others: internists, general practitioners, house officers, nurses, family members. Heroes ignore patients' subjective experiences of being unwell, unfit. Patients suffering from illness are frequently labeled "complainers" by heroic surgeons who, knowing they excised disease, resent the patients' unabated demands for care.

CAN A BAD PERSON BE A GOOD SURGEON?

What of character?

When asked to describe her ideal surgeon, a senior surgeon, after outlining the attributes of her two partners, spoke with reluctant admiration of another man: "Ross is a nasty son-of-a bitch—excellent surgeon, fantastic surgeon! Nasty to the patient, nasty to everybody. Do you know, that's not an ideal situation." The "nastiness" may have been less than ideal, but the man came to mind, when she was asked about her ideal surgeon.

Whether we believe healing is a part of a surgeon's mission will influence how essential a good character is to being a good surgeon. The technician does not have to use himself, as a person, to affect the welfare of the patient, as a person. If he is a good enough technician, his character is not central to his surgical competence.

This is perhaps an oversimplification. Painstakingness, willingness to take responsibility, and trustworthiness—coming through for the patient—are also aspects of character, as essential to curing disease as to healing illness. The surgical hero, then, cannot lack character. Some aspects of his character, however, may be less than admirable without disqualifying him as a hero. A surgeon may be nasty, uncaring, even venal, yet be brilliant in diagnosing and excising disease and managing postoperative care. Such a person might have great ability to care *for* the patient—without caring in the least *about* that patient.

The nasty, uncaring hero is the surgeon patients and critics of medicine abhor. Their complaints are justified. Nevertheless, such people may be good surgeons. Possibly, very good surgeons.

Not all heroes have poor characters. Many surgeons who define their mission as caring for patients' bodies, not their persons, are admirable human beings. They may care about their patients but define this caring as "personal," rather than as being an aspect of their professional role. And some heroes care deeply about their patients as persons. Comparing the brilliant technician with the hero who cares, whom he termed "the complete hero," the chief said: "The hero does dazzling and dramatic things and pulls them off successfully. The complete hero can be put in a full setting; not only does he have the talent and the power, but the character."

The "complete hero" is admired and loved by patients and their families and is honored and emulated by younger colleagues, who observe the effects of caring and learn the significance of healing from his interactions with patients. The complete hero is the Exemplary Surgeon; technical and moral excellence are joined. He is a good *surgeon*, and he is a *good* surgeon.

2

THE TEMPERAMENT OF SURGEONS

To be on the wire is life; the rest is waiting.

> Attributed to trapeze artist Karl Wallenda,
> on returning to the high wire after a
> fatal accident in his troupe

Yet there it was. *Manliness, manhood, manly courage . . .*
there was something ancient, primordial, irresistible
about the challenge of this stuff, no matter what a sophisticated and rational age one might think he lived in. . . .
A fighter pilot soon found he wanted to associate only
with other fighter pilots. Who else could understand the
nature of the little proposition (right stuff/death) they
were all dealing with? And what other subject could
compare with it? It was riveting!

> Tom Wolfe
> *The Right Stuff*

"BE BALLSY: DO IT!"

*S*URGEONS DISPLAY a specific and recognizable temperament, or ethos, "a standardized system of emotional attitudes"[1] that differs from that of members of other medical
specialties. The surgical ethos resembles that of the test pilots

trained as the first cadre of astronauts,[2] to whom several surgeons I interviewed in 1980 compared themselves.[3] The legendary Chuck Yeager, who walked away from demolished planes to become the first man to fly faster than the speed of sound, might well be the surgeon's heroic ideal. Like Yeager, the successful surgeon takes risks, defies death, comes close to the edge, and carries it off. Yeager's characterization of test pilots as "a breed apart" could have been uttered by a surgeon. (Modesty is not a surgical attribute; those who display "the right stuff" disdain those who do not.)

This chapter examines the temperament, or ethos, of those who perform surgical "miracles" and shows how it is related to the requirements of surgery. It then explores the price surgeons—and, on occasion, patients—pay for these traits, or emotional attitudes.

The surgical temperament (or standardized system of attitudes) is selected for when chiefs of surgery interview house officers. Self-selection is involved as well. Said one senior surgeon, "I liked [internal] medicine, but I didn't like the people in it; they were all . . . well, when I was a kid, they were the kind of kids I would have beat up!" (Surgeons frequently compare themselves to internists. The comparisons are always derogatory; on occasion they are presented as "jokes," but the underlying theme is serious: surgeons *act,* while internists merely think. Internists make similar invidious comparisons, but the evaluation differs: surgeons merely act, while internists take the time to think about what they're going to do before doing it. Naturally, the fact that I was married to an internist may have encouraged these disparaging remarks in my presence.)

Those who lack these attitudes, or traits, are unlikely to be attracted by surgery. If they enter a training program, they are likely to leave, voluntarily or involuntarily; and, if they remain, they are likely to be ill-suited to the practice of surgery. The temperament, or ethos, of surgeons is related to the "miraculous" attributes of surgery. Perhaps the most significant is *the relationship of surgery to time*. Recent writings have emphasized an understanding of medical care as a *process,*[4] with the passage of time perceived as an integral part of the interaction between doctor, patient, and disease. Surgery, however, unlike specialties such as internal medicine, is based primarily upon *event,* not process. Although processes, such as preoperative and postoperative care, vitally affect the outcome, the *act of surgery* occurs in a measurable and limited period of time. An operation does not unfold; it occurs. It is performed. The threat of death is always present. At the operating table, surgeons are rarely allowed the luxury of second thoughts; they cannot try a treatment, see if it works, augment or alter it, and then, if their first attempt is unsuccessful, try another approach. The surgeon must exhibit decisiveness, certitude, control; emergencies must be resolved, unexpected findings anticipated, small advantages exploited. Although every medical specialist enacts the metaphor of the "war on disease," for the surgeon, the encounter is more likely to be a battle than an extended war. Tactics, not strategy (to use von Clausewitz's distinction between conducting battles and wars), are primary, as the surgeon strives to extirpate disease, rather than attempting to outthink and outmaneuver it to slow its ravages. Says surgeon Richard Selzer: "The surgeon, armed to the teeth, seeks to overwhelm and control the body; the medical man strives with pills and potions to cooperate with that body. . . . One is the stance of the warrior; the other, that of the statesman."[5]

The advice of a chief resident to an intern might be emblazoned on a surgical pennant: "Be ballsy, do it!" Surgeons value decisiveness, confidence, nerve; they belittle internists, whom they describe as hesitant, indecisive types, who "sit on" gravely ill patients, rather than doing something, anything, to make that patient better.[6] A house officer gleefully narrated how he and other residents had removed a patient from an intensive care unit controlled by internal medicine, where they felt the man was getting inadequate and incorrect care; they just went and got him—"like a mugging"—and put him in the surgical intensive care unit, where they changed his "meds" [medications] and "lapped" him [performed an exploratory operation to see what was wrong]. "Not a mugging," said a senior surgeon, laughing, apparently unconcerned that the operation had found no operable disease: "search and destroy!" And, as a team prepared for an emergency operation on a young man who had swallowed lye for his second, or possibly third, suicide attempt, a chief resident, asked what he thought about operating on someone who might well go out and try again if the operation succeeded, responded: "I think he's twenty-six years old, and he's dying!"

During a portion of an operation, when a crucial artery was clamped and time was of the essence,[7] the senior surgeon directed the following exhortations to the chief resident, who was assisting him in joining a graft to the artery: "Take advantage! A surgeon has to be an exploiter. Exploit your advantage. You got too much against you! Anything you can do, you can get away with, will go much better. Run with the ball! Steal the case from me [work so rapidly and aggressively that you do all the difficult interesting parts before I get to them]. A chief resident has to run with the ball!" (He then remarked to the circulating nurse, whom he had criticized several times during the operation: "If you ran a bordello the way you ran the operating room this morning, you'd go out of business!" She responded, *sotto voce*, "I'd make a helluva lot more money. And I'd be off my feet!")

This surgeon's commanding, arrogant, egotistical approach, which he was trying by example and exhortation to convey to the resident, is perhaps extreme, but in no way unusual. "Decision making is so important in surgery, if you aren't possessed by a profoundly powerful ego, you couldn't stand it," said a chief of surgery, noting that the surgical motto is: "Sometimes in error, never in doubt." "I wouldn't be doing this if I didn't think I could help him," proclaimed a young orthopedist, carrying out a new and complex procedure. The nurse whispered that an old-time orthopedist had once announced, "All surgeons think they're the best; they wouldn't be here, otherwise!" In similar fashion, a chief resident, who agreed with me when I admired a particularly beautiful plastic [surgery] closing he had just completed, remarked, "They haven't made a humble surgeon yet!"

"Surgeons are involved in important things," said a chief. "They're decisive. . . . A guy who becomes a surgeon rather than an internist is a guy who needs a lot of positive, ongoing feedback. Every day the moment of truth occurs in the operating room, and that confirms he is right—right about the diagnosis, right about the timing, right about the procedure. . . . A surgeon can't stand a chronic patient. He likes to be able to define the patient's problem, do something definitive about it, and see that resolve the problem. The results are clear then, to the patient and to the surgeon."

Like the test pilot, the surgeon must have nerve. "Why does a surgeon need nerve?" I asked a young urologist. "Because we have to make snap decisions," he responded. He explained that a surgeon is constantly faced with the unexpected: something unexpected is found during an operation, or something unexpected occurs and the surgeon must decide instantly what to do. There's one surgeon at our hospital who lacks nerve, he said; he has technical skills but cannot make snap decisions. Consequently, he's slow, so slow that it's dangerous for his patients. Although he did not name this man, I had heard remarks and jokes about his slowness. The disastrous consequences of that slowness, however, were not yet apparent to me.

I asked a group of house officers, "Why does a surgeon need nerve?" "What do you mean, nerve?" inquired one. "What Dr. Sylva calls 'balls!'" responded another. "You need nerve to cut," he explained, eloquently describing the tension and excitement he feels when operating; his pulse, he said, goes from 70 to 135.

In describing the temperamental characteristics of surgeons and relating them to the "miraculous" attributes of surgery, I am not assuming a one-to-one correspondence. The attributes of operations overlap, as do the temperamental traits. I have isolated both for analysis; in reality, they shade into each other. The requirements of surgery call for a certain kind of person, however, and a rough correspondence exists between these attributes of operations and the temperamental traits of those who perform them.

Operations are *spectacular*. They contain an element of drama, theatre, spectacle. They take place in an "operating theatre"[8] under spotlights, performed in front of an audience by men who are "on stage." The results, too, can be spectacular: the patient was dying; the patient is cured. "The surgical panache!" said a chief, smilingly, when I mentioned surgeons' theatrical flair. Although temperamental differences exist, many surgeons are high-profile personalities; egotistical, arrogant, demanding, they take up a lot of psychic space.

Operations are *definitive and irreversible;* they change the body permanently. It is terrifying to cut into the human body, to alter it forever. "It is no small thing to dismember the image of God," said John Woodall, a sixteenth-century surgeon. "You have to be arrogant to be a surgeon," said a house officer. "It's a pretty arrogant thing to do to cut into tissue." Surgeons accentuate danger, challenge, bravery; their behavior and imagery are martial. "You have to approach an operation like a battle," said an orthopedist. "You have to know ahead what may go wrong and have three solutions planned for every problem." Surgeons delight in the hand-to-hand combat of the operating room: "A surgeon is never so happy as when he's operating," said a chief, singing tunelessly as he scrubbed for an operation. And, a senior resident remarked, after operating, "I was in such a bad mood, and now I feel good. I love to operate; it always makes me feel good!" When surgeons discuss operating, they sound like men describing why they love war.[9] "The intensity, the intensity . . . everything goes on tilt!" said a Vietnam veteran, discussing war. I suspect that operating, too, is intense, terrifying—and addicting—and that the everyday world seems drained and dull after the highly colored confrontation with death. "Time stops," remarked one man, describing operating. On the similarities between surgery and war, he declared, "Yes, in war, also, people get a name for themselves. You can *show* your bravery."

Operations, like miracles, are *attributable*. Everyone knows who performed it. Bad results are visible, blamable—and blamed. "In surgery there's nobody to blame a bad outcome on but yourself," said one man. "Unlike internal medicine, where they can blame it on the disease or the drugs, in surgery, the buck stops with the surgeon." Good results are equally visible and attributable. Many surgeons spoke of the "immediate gratification" of operating on someone and making them better fast. Surgeons may be blamed more than other specialists for bad results, but then, they are admired, praised—even adored—for good ones. A surgeon requires immediate, rapid, and positive feedback; the intellectual interest of the problem, in and of itself, is rarely enough. We might speculate that the kind of person who becomes a doctor is someone who likes to be admired, while the kind of person who becomes a surgeon is someone who *needs* to be admired. Performing a "miracle" may be as essential to the self-image of the surgeon as to the well-being of the patient.

Although the "miracle" is attributed to one person, the surgeon's war against death and disease is actually waged by a team. In this respect, the surgeon's performance differs significantly from the test pilot's solo flight. The surgical team is hierarchical, with an all-powerful commander, who directs the combat and accepts final responsibility for the outcome.

The team includes the anesthesiologist, two or more nurses, and a first, and on occasion second, assistant.[10] In a "teaching hospital," the assistants are likely to be house officers, who frequently perform the operation, guided by the senior, or attending, surgeon. The attending surgeon, whose patient is on the operating table, directs; he decides how much the senior house officer will do, how it will be done, and what to do if the resident gets into difficulties. He shows where to make the incision, what kind of incision to make, and what instrument to use for each procedure. Much of this is done nonverbally, with the "attending" holding instruments, helping, and indicating what should be done next. At the same time, junior house officers are taught how to hold retractors and perform simple procedures. The attending sets the mood in the operating room: he quizzes house officers, testing their surgical knowledge; commends or chastises the operating-room nurses; is serious, or decides it is time for joking (usually, when the patient is being "closed" after a successful procedure). "Good surgery is like good theatre," explained a senior house officer. "You can use your emotions to motivate the scrub nurse and the others." He then quoted from a Hippocratic aphorism: "The physician must not only be prepared to do what is right himself, but also to make the patient, the attendants, and externals cooperate."[11] Not surprisingly, one of the qualities chiefs of surgery seek in prospective house officers is "leadership ability." With hierarchy goes responsibility: a second-year house officer teaches and directs a first-year intern; the third-year resident teaches both; the chief resident teaches and directs all the house officers, and is in turn taught and directed by the attending surgeons. A solo performer would make a poor surgeon; it is not a one-on-one encounter.

Being a team player is essential, but the contest is brutal, and as the legendary football coach once said, winning isn't everything, it is the *only* thing. "Yes, he's good," said a senior surgeon of a house officer, "but I wish he were more *aggres-sive.*" "Mark would have made a good general surgeon," said a chief resident of an intern going into plastic surgery. "He's smart, aggressive, and a little bit of a son of a bitch." When asked why being a "son of a bitch" was useful, he explained, "Because you have to stand up for yourself sometimes and insist on doing things your own way."

Surgeons, like test pilots, display "the right stuff" in every area of life. The masculine society of surgeons admires cars, sports, speed, competence. "You drive like an internist!" said a chief of surgery, crushingly, to a female house officer who claimed it took longer than his estimate of two and a half hours to reach a distant city. The two nonsurgical subjects most frequently discussed at the surgeons' table in the cafeteria [12] were cars and sports. (I suspect that, in my absence, women were discussed in the same loving detail as sports cars, but this subject was downplayed when I was at the table. Later in the year, when I showed no disapproval, discussions of women occurred more frequently.) The sports were team sports: football, baseball, basketball, and occasionally, soccer. "Surgeons love the notion of teams pitted one against the other, or of single combat," testifies Selzer, adding, "It is fitting that this be so." [13] The women discussed were rarely wives; the young surgeons seemed to have an intensely polarized view of women, categorizing them into the kinds of women one married as opposed to the exciting "loose" women one played around with. "What's the female equivalent of 'stud'?" inquired an intern. After consideration, another house officer responded authoritatively, "Slut!" Many of the young surgeons talked about previous sports prowess, regretting that they now lacked the time to continue these activities. The chief, too, occasionally referred to his career in semiprofessional football. Reporting interviews with prospective house officers, he mentioned sports ability in tones of interest and approval. During thirty-three months of research, I heard enough operating-room discussions of intramural baseball games, where the surgeons had challenged the internists, to allow me to inquire with some confidence: "Surgery won?" They always had. (It was irrelevant whether or not the surgeons were better players: the internists had other things on their minds besides winning; the surgeons thought of nothing but winning.) I learned to distinguish surgeons from members of other medical specialties by their carriage and gait; surgeons walk with an upright, confident stride. A number of the surgeons I observed wore no overcoats, even in freezing temperatures; a coatless senior surgeon explained, only half-jokingly, "Surgeons are macho, cold doesn't bother us!" (Wondering which came first, the choice of surgery or the avoidance of overcoats, I asked an intern who was wearing only a cotton lab coat in below-zero weather, when he stopped wearing winter coats. "Since I was old enough to do it without my mother yelling at me," he responded.) The archetypal surgeon is invulnerable, untiring, unafraid of death or disaster. Of thirty-six general surgeons surveyed, eleven never wore automobile seat belts; six more reported that they reluctantly began to use them when a law mandating seat belts went into effect. Said one: "I resent them trying to force me to use them . . . it doesn't hurt anyone but myself." I was startled by the number of the surgeons I observed who smoked. I have no statistics, but I suspect a significant difference exists between the number of surgeons and members of other medical specialties who smoke.

Surgeons hold the image of the invincible hero who combats disease and rescues patients from death. During a complex and difficult operation, one said to a colleague: "You know that logo with Sir Lancelot, on a horse, carrying a sword? Well, we should have you on a horse, with a scalpel!"

The shadow image of the surgeon as hero is the "wimp." The wimp is not "ballsy." The wimp does not "do it." "What's all this wimpiness, you sound like an attending," said a house officer to a chief resident who advocated a more prudent course than the daring and risky actions he favored. Similarly, a general surgeon described a plastic-surgeon colleague whose hobby was making miniature furniture, as "a real wimp." "What did you do this weekend?" he inquired in a mocking tone of voice, responding in falsetto tones, "Oh, I just made itsy-bitsy furniture!" "Miniature furniture," he exploded, "the man's wimped out!" He told how *Road and Track* had rated this man's car as one for "effeminate men and butchy women—a wimp car," he concluded (he himself drove an Aston Martin). Later, this same man laughingly described a hospital party where a new director of surgery had dumbfounded his subordinates by bringing his wife. There were all the surgeons and house officers fooling around with women who were not their wives. Then, the director had arrived with his wife, and there *he* was, one of the director's senior surgeons, doing a slow bump and grind with a nurse pressed closely in front of him and another pressed to his back! Was he intimating that bringing one's wife to a surgical party was wimp behavior? This surmise was supported by the remarks of a nurse, who reported that the man whose hobby was making miniature furniture was one of the few surgeons in the hospital who was faithful to his wife. "Surgeons," said the possibly biased nurse, whose romance with a surgical house officer had just terminated, "seem to think they're entitled to the fastest cars, the showiest sports, the prettiest women."

The wimp is the symbolic inversion of the swashbuckling surgical hero. He is defined by what he is *not*. A wimp lacks nerve, daring, self-confidence, flair, machismo. A wimp does not display the martial virtues; he could never aspire to be a test pilot; he is fated to be ground crew (an internist, perhaps—or lower still, in a surgeon's estimation, a psychiatrist or pediatrician). A wimp wears an overcoat in cold weather and fastens his seat belts. Most important, a wimp lacks the supreme self-confidence that he, and only he, can walk into the operating room and save that patient's life.

I have related four "miraculous" attributes of operations (their rapidity, spectacularity, definitiveness, and attributability) to the temperament, or ethos, of those who perform them. I then showed how the *wimp* is the obverse, or symbolic negation, of this surgical temperament, or system of attitudes. We will now examine the final, most "miraculous," attributes of operations: successful operations have *an aspect of mystery, unpredictability, and wonder;* and *they are performed by someone with special powers.* Here, we move into another dimension, as we explore the ritual aspect of operations and the special relationship between surgeons and patients.

SURGERY AS RITUAL DRAMA

The religious antecedents of the metaphor of the miracle, and other metaphors I use in subsequent chapters, highlight a latent dimension of surgeons' relation to their work. Surgery is practical, it is technical, it is based upon knowledge, judgment, and experience—and yet, it also has an ineffable, transcendent aspect. Much of surgery can be described as a kind of ritual drama.

Although surgeons present themselves as simple men of action, who *do* rather than reflect or theorize, their "simplicity" covers a complex and nondiscursive attitude toward their occupation, their patients, and the human body whose secret recesses they disclose and violate. "To do surgery without a sense of awe," says Selzer, "is to be a dandy—all style and no purpose." [14] Selzer, who describes seeking the exact location of the soul in the recesses of the body and characterizes the surgeon as a priest, who gazes into the forbidden geography of the body, is more candid than his colleagues, many of whom, I am convinced, share his wonder and awe. The charismatic healer, endowed with gifts of grace, must believe in his powers in order to exercise them. This belief in one's special powers is also, I believe, a part of the surgical temperament. To explore surgery as ritual drama, let us begin with descriptions of two rituals of asepsis, the procedures that insure sterility by excluding microorganisms from an area.

Eileen, a surgical intern, and the operating-room nurses, taught the inexperienced anthropologist how to behave in the operating room. Imitating Eileen, I removed my clothes in the women's dressing room, put on a green cotton "scrub suit," covered my shoes with paper booties, my hair with a paper cap, and my face with a surgical mask. We then crossed the sterile portion of the OR (operating-room) suite (where everyone wore masks, caps, and scrub suits) to enter the operating room.

Respecting the Sterile Field

Field Notes. One of the nurses explained to me about the "sterile field." Between the instruments (which at the beginning were on the left of the patient, if one stood by the door) and the patient, was the sterile field; no one can go into it who is not scrubbed. One could walk on the right—and later, when the instruments on their table were moved to the foot of the patient—one could walk on either side of the patient. If you are not scrubbed, you should stay a foot away from someone who is scrubbed, and always face their front, so you don't accidentally back into them. (Their backs do not seem to be part of the sterile field, just their fronts.) The surgeons were scrubbed, two house officers, a medical student (at least I think it was a student, I had a lot of trouble recognizing people I didn't really know well, with all their hair covered, and wearing surgical masks), the chief [of surgery, who was operating], and an OR nurse [the "scrub nurse"], who handed them instruments. The anesthetist was not scrubbed, nor was another nurse [the "circulating nurse"], who handed things to the scrubbed nurse—she handed wrapped packages of instruments to the sterile nurse, with the first layer unwrapped so the sterile ["scrub"] nurse could take the package, unwrap it, and put the sterile instruments on her table to hand to the doctors.

Scrubbing

Field Notes. She [Eileen] showed me how to scrub, which I did with her. Very complex and ritualized. First the water, which you put on and off with your knee. The disposable sponge is in a plastic packet over the sinks; you clean under your nails with the pick provided for that [in the packet with the sponge]; throw it in the sink; wash your fingers and hands at least ten times each, including the sides of the fingers; both hands; then wash downward from the fingers with hands held upwards so the unsterile portion goes back toward the elbows. You scrub to the elbows ten minutes, said Eileen. Then, holding your hands in the air, you go into the OR, opening the door with your hip. The scrub nurse hands you a towel. One end is used for one hand, the other end for the other hand, making sure it touches nothing else. Then the nurse or two nurses puts you into a gown and pulls the sleeves on (the second time, I made the mistake of pulling the sleeves up with my hands, which made them unsterile, and they had to give me a new gown). Then gloves are pulled over your hands and over the sleeves of the gown. The gown is fastened on the inside back and on the top by the nurse, who then, holding the belt by a little tab, pulls it around you, so a sterile portion goes over the back. Then she tears off the tab she's holding, and you tie the belt with your sterile gloves. Sterile hands must be held above the waist or rested on the operating table, as opposed to unsterile hands, which are held behind one's back.

The ritual of scrubbing is so focal to surgery that, among surgeons, the term substitutes for operating. To indicate that they helped operate on a particular patient, house officers will say they "scrubbed" on that case. A surgeon who wishes to assist in an operation will ask, "May I scrub in?" And a surgeon who leaves a room where an operation is still taking place "scrubs out."

I am not the first observer to perceive operations as ritual processes. Using Van Gennep's classic description of ritual, Pearl Katz has analyzed the temporal progression and spatial divisions that govern modern surgeons' performances.[15]

A surgeon also described scrubbing as a ritual, despite its scientific rationale (to destroy bacteria that cause infections); he noted that most surgeons scrub for ten minutes, although scientific studies have indicated that two minutes is sufficient. When I told how a friend had observed operations in Russia, where these elaborate precautions were not followed, he responded that in the emergency room he sometimes operates in street clothes and things turn out pretty well. He continued his argument, describing the little window between the operating room and the sink area, where everyone in the operating room can watch the surgeon scrubbing, and the surgeon can look through and see everyone in the OR waiting for him. That window isn't really necessary, he declared, and yet, there it is, so everyone can look at the surgeon while they wait for him. It's a ritual, he proclaimed, like a religious ritual. When he was a house officer, he said, he noticed that the entire team of surgeons starts to scrub together, but, somehow, the intern walks into the operating room first, then the resident, and finally the senior surgeon. They always seem to walk in arranged by rank with the senior surgeon last.

"Surgery is a lot of ritual and a little science," said a female surgeon critically. "The boys need high mass, incense, and altar boys." [16] Perhaps it is not only "the boys" who need such rituals. The ritual is related, in part, to the mystery and unpredictability of operations.

✳

An element of uncertainty, of mystery, is always present in surgery. Although the statistical odds for particular procedures performed on particular diseases have been calculated, these probabilities aggregate operations, diseases, patients, and surgeons, as though each performance of a particular operation resembled the next; each case of a particular disease were identical to another; each patient, physiologically, biologically, and personally equivalent to the patient in the next bed; and each surgeon interchangeable with any of his colleagues. Because none is equivalent—*not even the same procedure performed by the same surgeon at two different times in the same day*—the statistics cannot predict what will occur on a specific occasion. In a probabilistic universe, the surgeon cannot be certain that even a comparatively routine procedure, such as a hernia repair, will not "go bad."

Ritual can allay anxiety,[17] propitiating the irrational and mysterious powers that control the odds. The anxiety, and the consequent insistence upon ritualistic procedures that may have little scientific basis, such as scrubbing for ten minutes rather than two, lend a magical quality to procedures many surgeons insist on.[18]

The act of surgery can be analyzed as a ritual drama, occurring in a "sacred" and secluded area, which is barred to the uninitiated. The surgeon who described scrubbing as a ritual pointed out that in ancient times, when terrifying procedures such as trepanning (cutting holes in the skull) were performed, the surgeon and the priest were the same person. He declared: "It's the ultimate intimacy, the ultimate power, putting them to sleep and playing with their insides, playing with their essence. The soul is in there somewhere, you know." Interestingly, in ancient Greek drama, which originated as religious ritual, performers also wore masks.

In this ritual drama, masked surgeons behave heroically,[19] in a special, secluded, ritual space. Wearing a distinctive costume that obscures his face and hair, the surgeon is, in some ways, most himself—or most the self he wishes to be. ("To be on the wire is life; the rest is waiting.") The surgeon is playing hero, "playing God," working miracles. Within the sacred space, life-and-death matters of high danger and heroism are enacted. These awesome and frightening characteristics of the ritual drama may disconcert critics, who wish to rationalize the charismatic powers of surgeons, transforming them into technicians—or butchers.

The ritual aspects of surgery and the priestly role of the surgeon, are as significant to the patient as to the surgeon. Surgery violates the integrity of the body; it penetrates the secret cavities, opens them to view, and alters the body irrevocably. After a lifetime of learning to protect our bodies, to avoid the pain and indignity of cuts and other infringements of inner space, we are then informed that this particular violation is necessary, that we must allow someone to dissect us and penetrate our inmost recesses. Not only the body but the psyche is injured; a sense of invincibility, inviolability, may be lost forever. "It's a scar on the body, it's a scar on the mind," said a house officer. Patients must have a very special relationship with someone whom they allow to penetrate their most secret recesses; the surgeons who violate the bodies must have a special relationship with the people whose bodies they penetrate. "It's a very close, intimate relationship with someone stripped of all their clothes, lying down in front of you so you can help them," said a chief of surgery. "It is only human love that keeps this from being the act of two madmen," says Selzer.[20] Those who enter these secret and protected recesses of the body inspire a sense of terror and awe,[21] but the feeling is profoundly ambivalent. Patients are conceding mysterious, terrifying, and extrahuman powers to people they know are only too human.

Performing surgery involves a dreadful power, that of life and death. Working a miracle is its positive aspect: doing something that rescues a person from death. "Playing God" is the negative aspect: the accusation hurled by angry and frightened patients and families, when surgeons refuse or are unable to perform a procedure that will save someone from death, or when they refuse to *stop* saving that person from an impending and inevitable death.

I heard few surgeons speak of this aspect of their profession. Surgeons prefer to present themselves as rational, technical men of science, with physical, not metaphysical, powers. (And yet, when I asked two exceedingly logical and matter-of-fact men whether they felt that surgery had a religious aspect, each said, "Yes, of course!" as though surprised that I should even bother to inquire.) I suspect surgeons rarely discuss the metaphysical aspects of surgery with each other. It's frightening to think of oneself as possessing such awesome power; it puts a heavy weight on someone who, however arrogant and egotistical, knows his abilities are fully—and merely—human.

THE PRICE: THE "PARANOIA" OF SURGEONS

During my first year of research, two unusually thoughtful and intelligent surgeons told me that surgeons, as a group, were "paranoid." What did they mean by "paranoid"? And why should surgeons be so described?

When asked to explain his use of the term, one man said that surgeons feel everyone conspires against them, to take patients away and find fault with their work. This "paranoia" is not a result of today's hostile climate, he contended; surgeons have always been like that. "Surgeons feel everyone's against them, even disease," explained the second. It gets worse as you get older, he continued; young surgeons, especially house officers, don't feel like this, because someone else is taking responsibility for the patient. You feel that way even when you don't get a patient, when a referring doctor sends a patient to someone else, said this surgeon, adding that his senior partner is like that. When an internist who refers a large number of patients to their group gives a patient to another surgeon, his partner goes *crazy;* he'll look at the chart and wonder what he did wrong.

Both surgeons spoke as though this paranoia were related to surgeons' belief in themselves. "Surgeons have tremendous egos," said the first. "They attribute every challenge to their judgment as a personal assault." The second surgeon explained, "You've got to believe you're the greatest to do what you do, you've got to feel you're gonna lick disease . . . and when it doesn't work, you ask what you or somebody else did to make things go wrong."

Let us examine this paranoia in action in the operating room:

"This is a really big operation, and yet they give me the smallest room in the place," remarked Dr. Verdi in a complaining tone, as he scrubbed his hands and arms with an antiseptic solution before entering the operating room, where the anesthetized patient was on the table. It *was* a big operation, and the family had replaced the young surgeon prepared to carry out the complex and time-consuming procedure with an older man, who divided his practice between this suburban community hospital and a celebrated hospital in the neighboring city. The patient's family had telephoned him on Sunday, said Verdi, to inquire about the results of tests carried out two days before. "Aren't you on call seven days a week?" they had asked, when Verdi wanted to know why they were calling on Sunday. A difficult family and a tricky case, he said, walking into the adjoining operating room.

"Sutton, you know when to give a case away!" he said sourly to the young surgeon who had been supplanted, but who observed and assisted during the first half of the operation. Later, another young surgeon, who came into the operating room to inquire how the case was going, commented, "This is a case where we used to say, 'Call the big boys!' " "Even the big boys are having trouble," responded Verdi, frowning. At one point, he jerked his left hand from deep within the patient, saying, "Ow, goddamn, I cut myself!" The younger man asked the nurses for an antiseptic and a new glove, saying, "He did it to himself, surrounded by enemies!" Later, when asked why his colleague had joked about his being surrounded by enemies, Verdi explained, "That's what I always say."

As Verdi carried out a particularly difficult maneuver, the younger surgeon groaned, "Oooh, that tweaks your testicles, that one," commenting admiringly when the maneuver was completed, "That was a bold move!" "That's because I had an audience," replied Verdi. Although he snapped once or twice at the chief resident who was assisting him ("Easy, Chuck, either you do the case or I do the case!") and got angry at one of the nurses, who was talking loudly to another nurse about something that had nothing to do with the operation ("I'm a temperamental surgeon," he said), Verdi talked and joked with his younger colleague and later described the course of events to another young surgeon, who dropped in to observe for a few minutes, and then with a colleague his own age, who strolled in to observe and comment.

Verdi directed the chief resident and Dr. Sutton, who was originally supposed to perform the operation, to feel a mass in the patient's abdomen. "Wow," said Sutton, "that might be severe benign disease!" "Well is it, or isn't it?" inquired the surgeon's contemporary, who had entered the operating room a second time. That was the question: was the mass malignant or benign? A sample of tissue had been sent to the pathology laboratory for analysis, but the pathologist wanted to examine more specimens before committing himself. "We're going to have to close him, whether it's benign or not," announced Verdi, explaining that the tumor was connected to too many internal organs to be removed. Meanwhile, the pathologist's feelings had been hurt; he thought he had heard laughter on the intercom from the pathology lab to the operating room. Verdi had to reassure him by telephone that no one had been laughing at him before the pathologist would announce that he had found cancer cells in the specimens.

Verdi called for a radiologist to pass a catheter to drain the patient's gallbladder (which could not be excised) and thus relieve the jaundice the patient was suffering from. The radiology resident, however, adamantly refused to insert the catheter until the next day. "When I get my next case, I'll take it to [the celebrated hospital in the city]," said Verdi. "I don't have to take all this abuse!"

He discussed draining the gallbladder with his contemporary, who returned with the younger surgeon to check on developments. "I would have put it [the catheter] in yesterday," Verdi said, "but the damn family's so difficult!" "There *is* no such thing as an easy family anymore," responded his colleague.

As he helped the chief resident sew the successive layers of tissue to close the incision, Verdi complained, "The whole damn world's against me!"

First, let me emphasize that although one might loosely use the term "paranoid" to describe aspects of this surgeon's style, Dr. Verdi is in fact an exceedingly sane, confident, successful man, highly respected by colleagues, admired and loved by patients. Verdi's remarks about the world being against him, exaggerated to the point of caricature, are presented as "jokes" and treated as such by the young surgeon who teased him about nicking his own finger. "Beleaguered" is another term we might use to describe his attitude of being surrounded by hostile forces.

What are the hostile forces against which the surgeon contends?

The most important are disease, and by extension, death. The surgeon's job is "to lick disease," and in this case, disease won. The patient's tumor was diagnosed as malignant and the surgeon was unable to arrest its spread by removing it. The term "malignant" assigns intention to cancer and, in fact, surgeons often behave—with cancer and other diseases, as well— as though locked in personal combat with a tricky, strong, and deceitful enemy.

Why is the surgeon's relationship with disease so personal? Two factors come to mind. The surgeon's victory is both attributable and visible. As noted, in surgery, victory is rapid, definitive, and ascribable to the surgeon. Moreover, surgery is a *public* act. It takes place before a limited and specialized audience (from which the lay public is rigorously excluded— unless cast in the role of patient, which involves being naked, horizontal, and anesthetized) composed of other professionals who also admire victory and note defeat. The public glory of victory is balanced by the fear—and shame—of public defeat. In addition to myself, eleven people observed all or part of this operation: the anesthesiologist; the chief resident; an intern;

two nurses; a third nurse, who successively relieved the others so they could have lunch; Dr. Sutton, the original surgeon on the case; a radiology resident, who came to discuss placing a catheter in the patient's gallbladder; a younger surgeon, who observed for a few minutes; another younger surgeon, who with his older partner, came in three times to observe and comment.

Surgeons know their performances are being observed and evaluated by a knowledgeable and critical audience. If not "surrounded by enemies," they are surely surrounded by observers, who are watching and judging. Moreover, each member of the audience may reenact performances with others: "bold moves" are described; errors in technique or judgment recounted; wins and losses calculated.

Four senior surgeons watched some part of the operation— Dr. Sutton, who had lost the case to an older, more experienced colleague, and three others. Everyone in the operating-room suite that day knew this was going to be a complex and challenging case; there had been talk of undertaking a particularly difficult and time-consuming procedure that was rarely performed at this community hospital. The bystanders may have been motivated by curiosity, friendship, or collegiality— also, perhaps by a certain competitive interest. Surgeons are competitive animals; perhaps the onlookers wanted to see how well this particular surgeon met this particular challenge. They wanted to savor his victory or, perhaps, his defeat. (The internist's victory, or defeat, is rarely as complete or attributable as the surgeon's, and it occurs in relative privacy.)

In addition to his observers, the surgeon has other elements to contend with. The people who schedule rooms, times, and assistants can help or hinder his work, and he often perceives them as hindering it. He wants an adequate operating room (not the smallest room in the place, where the staff and equipment necessary for a long and complex operation will be jammed together), proper scheduling (an operation that is likely to take a long time is best scheduled for the first thing in the morning, when everyone is fresh, not noon, or midafternoon, when nurses change shifts), a skilled anesthesiologist, good assistants (a capable and highly-trained first assistant, and for a complex procedure, a second assistant as well), experienced nurses, who keep their attention on the work (giving him what he asks for and having it ready even before he asks). In this case, the surgeon had to contend with a cranky pathologist, whose hurt feelings had to be soothed before he would analyze the specimens. The radiology resident was also recalcitrant, refusing to insert a catheter while the patient was on the operating table. Had the surgeon been able to remove the tumor and arrest the patient's disease, he might have overlooked these difficulties. Instead, he was defeated by disease, "abused" by pathologists, radiologists, and the head OR nurse (who scheduled operating rooms and times), and overlooked by nurses, who conversed with each other rather than anticipating his needs.

Another potentially hostile force was the patient's family. The surgeon perceived them as difficult and demanding. They had bypassed the young surgeon, who had been following the patient and was prepared to operate, telephoned a famous hospital in the neighboring city for names, and then asked this man, whose name they had obtained, to perform the surgery. They had called him on a Sunday to inquire about the results of a test performed on a Friday (about which they had been informed the day it took place). After the operation, he would have to talk with them, tell them that he was unable to remove the tumor and that "this tumor will kill him." Difficult families, tricky cases, and operations that do not result in a cure, add up to trouble. And in the stories surgeons tell one another in the operating-suite lounge, "trouble" consists of six-million-dollar lawsuits against surgeons with "only" one million dollars of malpractice insurance, whose fault was to lose the battle against disease and death.

Among the forces against which the surgeon feels he must contend, then, are disease, which the surgeon battles in a very personal, even personified form; the possibility of defeat, where instead of his "licking" disease, disease may lick him; the public character of his battle, and consequently defeat, with his "public" composed of those who are qualified, and perhaps eager, to pass judgment upon his performance; his dependence upon others, who may hinder his efforts (anesthesiologists, pathologists, radiologists, house officers, nurses); and the patient's family, who may love a winner but sue a loser. All these may be described in psychiatric terms as "reality factors." At least one is culture-specific: American patients and their families sue their physicians far more frequently than their British or Canadian counterparts. As a result, American doctors may perceive families, in part, as potential enemies, poised to sue if they do not get a good result ("There *is* no such thing as an easy family, anymore"). But there is more to it.

The surgeons who identified this "paranoia" in the first place spoke as if it were related, in some way, to surgeons' certitude, to their intense belief in themselves. How can this be?

In a celebrated essay entitled "Training for Uncertainty," sociologist Renée Fox describes how medical students are trained to deal with the basic uncertainties of medical practice.[22] These uncertainties, always present in medicine, result from imperfect mastery of knowledge, current limitations in that knowledge, and difficulty in distinguishing between personal ignorance and the current limits of medical knowledge. In a subsequent essay, Fox notes the mechanisms students used to cope with uncertainty, observing: "Students gradually evolved what they referred to as a more 'affirmative attitude' toward medical uncertainty. . . . In clinical situations, they were more prone to feel and display sufficient 'certitude' to make decisions and reassure patients."[23]

Another commentator, Jay Katz,[24] who is both psychiatrist and lawyer, interprets Fox's material differently. He notes that the medical students described by Fox exhibited increasing certainty as their schooling proceeded. Instructors encourage this certainty, he observes, by criticizing students when they display too much unsureness and indicating that doubt will make them less effective with patients. Katz suggests that medical education involves *"training for certainty,"* not uncertainty. This begins in medical school, being reinforced by postgraduate and specialty training. Interestingly, Katz's examples of what he considers dogmatic "certitude" involve surgeons.

I have noted that the surgical ethos stresses decisiveness, control, confidence, and certitude, and that these characteristics are selected for in surgical training programs and reinforced during that training. I have argued that these are necessary, that a person who is insufficiently decisive, certain, and in control is likely to make a poor surgeon.

Yet, in surgery, as in the other medical specialties, uncertainty remains. No one can command all the surgical skills and knowledge; knowledge itself falls short—there are questions no surgeon today can answer; and, surgeons may have difficulty distinguishing between their own lack of skills and knowledge and the limitations of present knowledge. Moreover, all of medicine is based upon statistical probabilities, and the application of the laws of probability to specific cases is always filled with uncertainty.

This tension between certainty and uncertainty may be stronger and more stressful among surgeons, who must manifest an overwhelming self-confidence to be effective in the operating room. The more certitude surgeons exhibit, the more troubling their inevitable feelings of uncertainty must be. A house officer explained: "You have to feel like a god, or act like a god. You have to believe that you know what's the best thing for the patient. Besides, the people with the most faith have the most doubts. When you read the lives of the saints, the closer they came to perfect faith, the greater their doubts."

Hence, the paranoia. A classic description of "paranoid

style" discusses the "suspicious thinking" characteristic of this mode.[25] The author points out that central to the understanding of paranoid style, pathology, and symptoms is the mechanism of projection: *"the attribution to external figures of motivations, drives, or other tensions that are repudiated and intolerable in oneself."* [26]

What I am suggesting is that surgeons, who must display control and certitude to presume to "dismember the image of God" may attribute their feelings of uncertainty *to others,* who are perceived as conspiring against them. The certainty can then be perceived as an inner state, related to the surgeon's confidence and competence, while the uncertainty is blamed upon outside forces, those who hinder and find fault with his work.[27]

We can then understand why this paranoia might increase as a surgeon grows older. The greater his reputation and responsibility, the greater the demands on a surgeon to exhibit certainty; the greater the doubts he must defend himself against; and the more strongly he may project those doubts outward, perceiving them as caused by the behavior of others. If "you've got to believe you're the greatest to do what you do, you've got to feel you're gonna lick disease," then when disease wins, you retain certitude by inquiring what *somebody else* did to make things go wrong.

The paranoia may be an inevitable corollary of the control and certitude necessary to dismember and permanently alter the image of God in the surgeon's battle against disease and death.

THE PRICE FOR PATIENTS

If indeed surgeons exhibit a special temperament, or ethos, being activist, egocentric, decisive, and confident to the point of arrogance, then we must realize that patients, too, may pay a price when they relate to such persons. I have noted that the examples of dogmatic certainty cited by Jay Katz involve surgeons.[28] Some of the behavior that Katz and other medical critics call for from doctors, including acknowledging uncertainty and giving patients a greater voice in decision making, may be particularly difficult for people with the "surgical temperament." The lack of this kind of support is the price the patient may have to pay for a "miracle worker."

If we believe that the surgical temperament is useful and adaptive in the operating room, we may also be forced to recognize that this particular price for patients is necessary. It may be the exceptional surgeon who is capable of recognizing and supporting the autonomy of patients, of allowing them to share decision making, of acknowledging uncertainty in the face of decisions that must be made. Such people surely exist, but perhaps we cannot expect them to be the temperamental or behavioral norm among surgeons.

3

THE FELLOWSHIP OF SURGEONS

> By primary groups, I mean those characterized by intimate face-to-face association and cooperation. They are primary in several senses but chiefly in that they are fundamental in forming the social nature and ideals of individuals.
>
> Charles H. Cooley
Social Organization

> *Fellowship.* Everyman, good morrow, by this day!
> Sir, why lookest thou so piteously?
> If any thing be amiss, I pray thee me say,
> That I may help to remedy.
>
> Anonymous
Everyman and Medieval Miracle Plays

IN THIS chapter, I examine the relationships among senior surgeons who work at the same hospital(s), see each other several times a week, hear about each other's successes, failures, scenes, and situations more often than that; surgeons who, among each other, may fight, play ferocious practical jokes, relay gossip and scandal, steal patients, yet join together when threatened by outsiders, be they hospital administrators, litigious patients, critical laypersons, or members of other specialties. Within this small group, admiration, ridicule, and the attribution of roles becomes a kind of communal "morality play" that operates to regulate the behavior of members. There is, however, a price for this kind of community.

THE FELLOWSHIP

I am not sure just how to refer to the face-to-face group of surgeons who operate in the same hospital. I have used the term "fellowship" in its medieval senses of "a community of interest, sentiment, nature"; "the members of a corporation or guild"; or "the body of fellows in a college or university; the society constituted by the fellows,"[1] although these definitions do not suggest the geographic basis for the association. Various anthropological and sociological concepts are also relevant: "community," "primary group," and "network" might also be used to describe this group.[2] The term "community" is apposite if we think of it as describing a *relationship,* rather than a specific and limited geographic location. The fellowship, or community, of surgeons can be identified by the following characteristics:

1. *It is recognized by members, who perceive themselves as belonging.*

Attending surgeons at a hospital know one another, and whether or not they like each other, they perceive themselves as a group set off from, say, the internists at that hospital, whose behavior they describe by a series of jokes and disparaging remarks.[3] "The relationship between surgeons is very different from the one between medical doctors," said a chief of surgery. "We may fight like hell, but we join together if we're threatened by anyone else." Unlike the "little community"[4] cherished by traditional anthropology, however, the community of surgeons is not neatly bounded: a surgeon may operate at two or more hospitals

and consequently belong to several such groups.[5] In this respect, the grouping is closer to the concept of a "network."[6]

2. *Members have frequent face-to-face contact.*

Surgeons encounter one another in the OR suite. They
change from business suits to "greens" (scrub suits) together in the men's locker room. They may scrub side by
side at separate faucets in the same long sink or stop to
joke and chat with colleagues who are scrubbing. Friends
occasionally drop in on one another's operations to observe, comment, and advise; members of the same surgical
practice group may "scrub in" and help a partner. Between operations, surgeons sip coffee in the OR lounge and
"schmooze" with colleagues. No one can predict the exact
duration of an operation, so that subsequent operations
slated for that operating room frequently take place later
than the time listed on the OR schedule. As a result, a
surgeon scheduled to operate in a particular room at a
particular time may have to wait for the previous surgeon
to finish. Moreover, unscheduled emergencies occur, and
surgeons and operations can be "bumped" to make room
for an emergency procedure.

Surgeons may encounter colleagues while dictating
postoperative notes[7] or looking in on patients in the "recovery room," where patients stay until their condition has
stabilized sufficiently to move them to the "unit" (the intensive care unit) or the "floor" (the surgical wards). They
see each other in the "unit" or on the "floor" while making
daily or twice-daily "rounds" on hospitalized patients.
They encounter one another in the cafeteria, grabbing a
cup of coffee or a snack between operations—or before
leaving to make rounds at another hospital. Some join
house officers and colleagues at the "surgeons' table" to
gossip and talk shop. They meet at the hospital's weekly
surgical M and M (mortality and morbidity) conference
and at grand rounds.[8] Every surgeon does not attend every

M and M conference but the surgeon involved is usually present when his patient is being discussed. Senior surgeons and house officers sign a list that is passed around; someone who misses too many meetings will be threatened with the loss of his "privileges" (the right to operate at a hospital).

3. *A collegial, peer relationship prevails; even when seniors have some authority over junior attendings, the ideology of collegiality holds.*

   The fellowship of surgeons resembles, in certain respects, the medieval "company" or guild. Members share similar training, an oath (the Hippocratic), and a presumed dedication to the welfare of their patients. As Freidson and Rhea note, doctors perceive themselves as "a company of equals."[9] Naturally, some members are more equal than others. The chief, for example, occupies a special interstitial role, representing the hospital's administration to surgeons and the surgeons to the administration. Although *as chief* he has authority over his colleagues, *as a surgeon*, he is regarded as a peer, being judged (and respected or disdained) by colleagues on his surgical abilities. In surgical practice groups, one person—most frequently the founder—is generally senior. It is he who selects his younger colleagues; he may employ them on a salaried basis before making them partners, and some may remain permanently salaried. This senior is given latitude about the operations he chooses to perform (see Chapter 6), the duration and timing of his vacations, and the evenings and weekends he chooses to be "on call" (available for patients' phone calls and emergencies). Nevertheless, in this situation as well, the *ideology of equality* prevails.

4. *Members have direct and indirect knowledge of colleagues' behavior.*

   In the operation described in Chapter 2, eleven people, in addition to the anthropologist, observed all or part of the procedure: an anesthesiologist; three house officers (two surgeons and one radiologist); three nurses; and four colleagues. All talk. All contribute to the hospital "grapevine." "If you make a mistake," said one surgeon, "it flashes around the hospital so quick that it's probably better to go out and grab the microphone and say, 'Hear ye, hear ye, this is Chuck Kurtz, I just cut the ureter!'" (a serious and unmistakable error).[10] I shall explore some of the functions of gossip below, but let me note here that surgeons know a great deal about their colleagues' actions during specific operations and about their behavior generally. Their knowledge may be based more upon hearsay than direct observation, but it exists. One surgeon, when asked for a technical explanation of the behavior of a colleague during a procedure about which house officers had expressed disquiet, swore me to silence before saying:

That guy's a disaster! He's intelligent, a "good operator" [has good operating technique]. But the house officers were right about the case the other day. The patient should have had those lines in her ahead of time, the arterial and Swan-Ganz, so they could have had a baseline reading. His [the surgeon's] saying some patients should have those things put in under anesthesia is just an excuse. The only reason she didn't is that [he] was too busy elsewhere. He does so many cases in so many places he just doesn't have time to take care of his patients. That guy's a disaster! I've had patients whom I've told they didn't need an operation and then they've gone to him for a second opinion and the next thing you know, they were booked as an "emergent" [emergency] case and operated on!

The surgeon mentioned two cases this colleague had scheduled for that day. In one, a vascular procedure was being performed on a patient's leg before the leg was amputated. He exploded: "That's garbage! The fem-pop [the vascular procedure] doesn't need to be done! And he's got an abdominal aortic aneurysectomy scheduled—that patient came in yesterday. The patient should have come in earlier for a major procedure like that to get a bowel prep.[11] He'll say the patient got it outside, but it won't be true!" The revelation, of one surgeon telling me, an outsider, about another surgeon's misbehavior, was rare, but I believe the knowledge of colleagues' doings and misdoings is common. A young surgeon, discussing an older colleague, told me that the man was not good at operating and had a bad reputation; the surgeon described how, during a colon operation, this man had severed the superior mesenteric artery [the blood supply to the colon], and over the house officers' objections that the colon was a "funny color," insisted everything would be fine; he had "closed" the patient, who then died. When you do something like that, said the young surgeon, there's no keeping it quiet; everyone hears about it, and you get a really bad reputation. Nevertheless, the young surgeon's partner, who also told me that this man had a bad reputation without giving any details, related how, when a hospital where this colleague was seeking privileges [to operate] had inquired about him, the surgeon had responded, with literal truthfulness, "I never shared an operating room with him; I don't know how good he is".[12]

This knowledge, of colleagues' behavior and misbehavior, spreads. Many surgeons operate at more than one hospital; house officers may be trained at several.[13] As a result, information about surgeons may circulate to colleagues who may not know the man on a daily, face-to-face basis. The man has a reputation; his ascribed role in the surgeons' "morality play" (to be discussed) may move beyond the confines of the hospital(s) where he operates.

5. *Members are profoundly concerned about colleagues' evaluations of their competence and character.*

I have little *direct* evidence to support this contention; surgeons rarely discussed the misbehavior of colleagues with me, or how they felt about the evaluations of their colleagues. They did, however, on occasion say that they admired someone, and when questioned, described what characteristics they found admirable. They also questioned me closely about colleagues' opinions of *them*. "Did he say anything about me?" some would demand with anxiety or elaborate casualness after I had spent a day following a colleague. Some responded to criticism I had *not* repeated, as though they wondered whether I had heard it—or as though that criticism played in their consciousness, like a musical tape or phonograph record. At surgical M and M's, I heard men react strongly to the judgments of peers, defending themselves fiercely and looking upset and depressed when colleagues suggested, however obliquely, that they had done the wrong thing for a patient. A few defended themselves to me afterwards, justifying the behavior that had been questioned and undermining the credibility of the colleague who had questioned their course of action. Moreover, on any number of occasions, I heard surgeons assert that outsiders—laypersons, patients and their families, even internists—were unable to understand, and consequently evaluate, their behavior. The implication was clear: only surgeons (especially colleagues, who understood the personal, social, and professional forces that constrained their actions) could judge surgeons.

I have not encountered another description of this fellowship, or community, of surgeons. Surgeons often talk as though they were Sir Lancelot, riding through the forest (followed, perhaps, by a squire) in a lonely quest for glory and renown—or the Lone Eagle, winging it across the Atlantic; critics often describe surgeons in similar fashion. Three ethnographers have studied general surgeons.[14] Charles Bosk[15] investigated surgical house officers in a public hospital with no private attendings; the two services he concentrated on each had two "full-time" attendings. Either the fellowship of surgeons did not exist at his hospital, or Bosk did not concentrate on it, as such. Marcia Millman observed various medical specialties in three hospitals. Although the title of her book, *The Unkindest Cut*,[16] suggests that her subject is surgeons, her examples (such as her description of the M and M conference) frequently refer to members of other specialties. Moreover, Millman focuses primarily on bad behavior by individuals, indicating how it is ignored or "neutralized" by the group, rather than focusing on the group itself. Pearl Katz[17] followed six senior surgeons for several weeks each in one hospital; if she noted the fellowship or community of surgeons, she did not describe it.

This relationship between surgeons involves informal, interstitial behavior. To observe the fellowship, to even become aware of it, the field-worker must "hang around" senior surgeons and house officers, tuning in to stories, veiled allusions, gossip, jokes. To study the fellowship in depth, a researcher probably requires access—as only Bosk had—to the men's locker room. I missed a great deal—as, I believe, do women surgeons, who change for operations in the nurses' (or women's) locker room.

In any case, surgeons know a great deal about the professional competence and moral rectitude of colleagues at their hospital and in their area. This information is transmitted through gossip and jokes and encapsulated in a series of role attributions in what, using a medieval analogy, I think of as a surgical morality play.[18]

INFORMAL LEARNING DURING TRAINING

Before we examine gossip and the cast of characters in the surgeon's morality play, let us briefly consider the training of surgical house officers and the informal mechanisms that impress upon them what kind of behavior is admired and what behavior is disesteemed.[19]

No definitive answer has been framed to the question of whether house officers are (as many of them contend) underpaid and absolutely essential employees, or (as many of their seniors believe) a kind of advanced student. If we think of the house officer as an *apprentice*, however, the two notions are not necessarily antithetical; the house officer is, then, doing necessary work while learning a profession.[20] Being an apprentice is a role or position; apprenticeship is also a *method of learning*. One learns by observing and doing—or, as the mocking aphorism about mastering a new procedure has it: "See one, do one, teach one."[21]

Apprentice surgeons learn more than procedures. They absorb skills, behaviors, values—some of which are manifest, some latent; some of which they know they are learning, some of which they learn without realizing it. The surgical ethos— "a standardized system of emotional attitudes"[22]—is acquired at this time. To be a competent surgeon, book learning—or "academics"—is necessary but not sufficient (see Chapter 1). Other essential, possibly nondiscursive, skills and values must also be absorbed. The novice acquires technical and clinical skills,[23] moral standards, social knowledge, and behavior.

These skills, abilities, and values are acquired not only through formal instruction; novices also learn through emulation or modeling. Said one young surgeon, describing a resident about three years ahead of her in the program where she was trained:

> [He] was the epitome of the macho surgeon, always running around, always overwhelmingly caring for his patients, almost to a fault, twenty-four hours a day, seven days a week in the hospital; there was nothing about his patients that he did not know, nothing ever, even the most small detail, went unattended to. I had a lot to do with him when I was a medical student and a junior resident and a lot of what I wanted to be was to kind of model myself after him. . . . In general, he was acknowledged to be one of the best residents ever in the program, and I thought if I could be like him, that wouldn't be such a bad thing.[24]

Novices emulate admired house officers and attendings, those they observe at work, and those who actively befriend them. In medicine, the role of the mentor, who befriends the young physician, teaching skills and behaviors, is vital. Novices model themselves upon their mentors consciously and unconsciously.[25] An academic "full-time" surgeon in his forties, who described how his mentor had trained him, advised him, and made sure he joined the right prestigious surgical societies, told how he had ignored his father's urgings to stop smoking but had abandoned the habit after receiving a letter from his mentor asking him to do so. A surgeon in his sixties described how he would invite promising house officers home for dinner and to his country place for weekends; he taught them how to behave, he said. Such social "fathering" may be particularly helpful to a young man whose brains and abilities have moved him several rungs up the social ladder (as, indeed, they had for many of the surgeons I studied). The father-son, mentor-student relationship is woven into the fabric of medicine: the Hippocratic oath requires the physician to take filial responsibility for his "adoptive father's" welfare.[26]

Admired behaviors, then, are acquired through formal instruction and practice, and, less formally, through observation and emulation. Knowledge about disparaged behaviors is also acquired through formal instruction, practice, observation—and ridicule.

When a house officer commits an error, the results can be serious, even fatal. As Bosk's study emphasizes, technical errors committed by surgical house officers are corrected and forgiven—provided the resident does not make the same error repeatedly.[27] What Bosk mentions only tangentially, however, is the ferocious "joking" the house officer is subjected to for weeks or possibly months. In one hospital I observed, an attending surgeon presented annual awards to residents for disesteemed characteristics, such as "Hands of Wood," "Marble Mitts," "Captain Blood" (to a house officer, who did not control patients' bleeding sufficiently), and to a junior resident who administered too much insulin to a diabetic patient, the "Claus Von Bulow Award." Such humor is entertaining only when a community is so closely knit that everyone knows exactly what behavior each award refers to. In Bosk's book about the training of house officers, an attending surgeon, Dr. Arthur, describes how, as a house officer trying to be helpful during a colon resection, he was accidentally responsible for bathing the open peritoneal cavity with liquid feces [which contain microorganisms that can cause serious infections]. From then on, reported Dr. Arthur, that particular maneuver was known as "the Arthur phenomenon."[28] Naturally, every time "the Arthur phenomenon" was mentioned, young Dr. Arthur writhed and recalled his error. His peers also remembered it—and were probably relieved the maneuver was named after Arthur, not them. Ridicule is a powerful stimulus to self-monitoring.

Although couched as a "joke," such ridicule cuts perilously close to the bone. I observed an operation where a young attending surgeon directed a stream of "joking" critiques to a house officer whose operating technique—his hemostasis [control of bleeding] in particular—the attending deplored. Before the procedure, the attending said to me: "If I had known he was scrubbing with me, I would have ordered two units of blood!" During the operation he addressed the following remarks to the resident and the room at large: "You haven't missed one yet [a little vein, such as the one the house officer had just severed], you turkey!" . . . "He's got seeing-eye scissors for 'bleeders' [a blood vessel that bleeds because it has not been closed by tying or cauterizing]." When, at another point in the procedure, the house officer said, "I don't want to cut off the blood supply," the attending rejoined, "He really knows about the blood supply, I can tell you that!"

House officers, then, learn admired and disesteemed behaviors in part through emulation and disparagement. Ferocious teasing of juniors by seniors helps teach the juniors not only what *not* to do but also a disciplined alertness, a concentration of attention and energy.

Similar mechanisms influence senior surgeons. With seniors, however, the "jokes" and disparaging remarks are expressed behind the surgeon's back. During an operation, a house officer said (naming a surgeon who was not present), "That's a Volpi cecum," and the attending, looking pointedly at me, cautioned: "Hush, no names!" The critical allusion is similar (the "Arthur phenomenon," the "Volpi cecum"), but the status of the speakers differs. Derision is expressed directly by superiors, indirectly by juniors and peers. Teasing becomes gossip. I heard the following exchange about a man whose slowness in operating was legendary in his hospital:

> *First surgeon:* "It takes him seven hours to cancel an operation!"
>
> *Second surgeon:* "When he begins to operate, they put away the clock and put up a calendar!"

Among "a company of equals," gossip helps enforce group standards and mark deviations from these standards.

Gossip has another function: it helps maintain the unity of groups and sets them off from outsiders.[29] As anthropologists thrust into strange milieux discover, to be able to gossip "properly," one must know the personnel and their histories, one must have enough technical and social knowledge to pick up veiled allusions, and one must be considered enough of an insider so that members are not insulted if one joins in. Gossip, then, does not only assert the values of the fellowship or community of surgeons; it helps create and maintain that fellowship.

THE MORALITY PLAY

Some of the information contained in gossip and admiring comments is encapsulated in certain roles, which are attributed to certain people. Every hospital seems to have an almost invariant cast of surgical characters: the Prima Donna, the Old-Time Surgeon, the Sleazy Surgeon, the Buffoon, the Compassionate Young Surgeon, the Exemplary Surgeon. They act in a contemporary species of the medieval morality play, whose cast of characters personifies various surgical virtues and vices. Surgeons refer to only two of these roles, or characters, by name: the Prima Donna and the Old-Time Surgeon. Although it was I who named the other characters, I am convinced that surgeons would recognize them. When I discussed the cast of characters with a chief of surgery, he agreed with the notion and the roles. I'll quote his comments as I present each character.

The first character who would be noticed by an outsider in a department of surgery is the Prima Donna. He has a very high profile. Bosk's description of a Prima Donna was recognized by several men with whom I discussed his book.[30] "Every hospital has one!" said a surgeon, with amusement. The Prima Donna "typically drives the chief nuts," said my informant, the chief of surgery. "He says 'I am not subject to peer review because *I* have no peers!' All departments of surgery are inhabited by prima donnas," he continued. "It's just that *the* Prima Donna is outstanding among them."

Bosk's description[31] suggests that the Prima Donna and the Old-Time Surgeon are the same person, and my early research bore this out. The chief of surgery, however, distinguished the two roles. He suggested that, while larger hospitals might contain the entire cast, smaller hospitals may have just some of the characters. Observation confirmed the chief's distinction between the Prima Donna and the Old-Time Surgeon. Not all Prima Donnas are older surgeons; some are young (Raoul, the chief resident who performed "another miracle" [page 1] is flamboyant and temperamental). And not all Old-Time Surgeons are theatrical; some are relatively low-key. Many Old-Time Surgeons, however, are (or were) full-blown Prima Donnas. "The Old-Time Surgeon thought he was king of the OR [operating room]," said an anesthesiologist. His theatrical display expressed dominance and helped to enforce instant, unthinking obedience. I have heard stories of Old-Time Prima Donnas who threw trays filled with instruments across the operating room when instruments or events were not to their liking. When asked if Dr. Sylva (see Chapter 6), an Old-Time Prima Donna, hurled trays, a long-term internist colleague responded: "He used to throw trays, in his time. He doesn't anymore." Perhaps one reason surgeons now refrain from such behavior in the operating room is that contemporary nurses are less obedient (less efficient, say older surgeons; less subservient, rejoin younger nurses). Today when nurses find a surgeon's behavior dangerous or inappropriate, they file an incident report, a formal written complaint, which, traveling up the administrative chain of command, may result in a reprimand or more serious sanction. An anesthesiology resident described how a surgeon at his hospital threw an instrument once and was told he would lose his privileges (permitting him to operate at that hospital) if he were to do so again.

The surgeon of yesterday, said one man, was almost a pioneer: everything he did was done almost for the first time; he had to be individualistic and resourceful. He said regretfully, "Instead of being the individualistic tough guy he used to be, today we have a swarm of technicians who come in with their lawyers and accountants and try to lock up a community." [32] Perhaps the temperament and situation of the Old-Time Surgeon was closer to that of Sir Lancelot or the Lone Eagle than is the surgeon of today.

My informant, the chief, distinguished the Buffoon, who hates it when everyone laughs at him, from the Clown, who, when everyone laughs at him, laughs with them. (I encountered no Clowns, but my experience is less extensive than the chief's.) Of the Buffoon, he said he's "a guy like the one in 'Li'l Abner' who walked around with a cloud over his head.

Every time something went wrong, you knew who was in back of it." The Buffoon is technically inept and has poor clinical judgment (for a discussion of technical skills and clinical judgment, see Chapter 1). A Buffoon makes *technical* errors;[33] it is the Sleazy Surgeon who makes moral errors—although the Buffoon's continuous string of technical errors, without either learning better or leaving surgery for another branch of medicine, might be perceived as a kind of moral error. I learned that a surgeon can be cast as Buffoon at one hospital, while at another, where he also operates, the role may be attributed to another actor. It is conceivable that, to be cast as Buffoon, a surgeon must possess not only technical and judgmental ineptitude but also an enemy or antagonist, a colleague who vociferously ridicules him behind his back and points out his deficiencies to others.

Of the Sleazy Surgeon, who cuts moral corners, my informant remarked:

> He's a trickster. He's very slick, he's very clever. . . . Characteristically, he has an incredible ego. Often he's a psychopath or sociopath. . . . That guy typically snows referring doctors, snows patients, even though he may ridicule them in their absence. He's a 'good operator'; he knows what his limitations are. He's usually involved with unnecessary procedures, although he covers his tracks. But he does operate with very few criteria to determine whether they [the procedures] should be done. For that reason, he's pretty hard to nail. He has to be very smart. If he's not smart, he will just get nailed, so he's got to have all the parts [brains, operating ability, and so on]. He tends to stay out of situations where he'll blow his cover. He does only what he can do well, and he's usually pretty talented, so in different situations he tends to do pretty well.

The man whose colleague described him as "a disaster" is a Sleazy Surgeon. So is a young man I observed, who managed to perform in the operating room a large number of procedures on nursing-home patients that his more scrupulous colleagues carried out, at a far lower rate, at the nursing home itself. One unfortunate diabetic patient, on whom Dr. X had performed five or six procedures, including amputating both legs—after the man had been rejected as too much of an operative risk by a surgeon in a renowned hospital—was referred to by a house officer as "Dr. X's meal ticket."

(I have less data on Buffoons and Sleazy Surgeons than I would wish. These are subjects that were rarely discussed in front of me; I'd hear bitter jokes and veiled remarks, but the subject would change if I asked questions, took notes, or even looked too interested. On occasion, someone—a house officer, nurse, or senior surgeon—would erupt with anger and frustration in front of me, or publicly characterize someone else's behavior as "sleazy." Most of my information is compiled retrospectively from my field notes, where I recorded jokes, remarks, and behavior that I did not understand at the time.)

Of the Compassionate Young Surgeon (see Chapter 5), the chief of surgery, with whom I discussed the Cast of Characters said: "He's the one the residents all warm to the most. He's always a conscientious and competent young surgeon. The residents spot him. He's always in a position where you can't fault his motives: he takes care of others' interests rather than his own." He named the man who filled the role at the celebrated hospital where he was trained and said that the nursing staff called this surgeon "Gentle Ben."

The Exemplary Surgeon, the man who is asked to operate on other doctors' families, is admired by house staff and colleagues. When I mentioned that I had never heard a bad word about one particular surgeon, a chief resident responded, "Yes, he has judgment, knowledge, character, and skill!" I noted that even the hospital Prima Donna deferred to this man, and the resident agreed, reporting that the Prima Donna yells at other surgeons, even the chief, but never yells at this man. "It's as though there were only two lions, with lots of other animals," he said. "They treat each other with respect and don't mess with one another." When I asked the surgeons of the same hospital whether any man there typified their ideal, several mentioned this man. A colleague (who belonged to a competing surgical group) gave his name, saying: "He has good academics, good background, looks the role, has good technical ability, cares for the folks. If I was going to model myself after someone, it would be him."

The most common role in the surgical cast of characters, said my informant, the chief, is "a good journeyman surgeon, who doesn't get into trouble and doesn't stand out, but takes good care of patients." This particular character might be named "Everyman."[34] The focal actor in the morality play, he hopes to behave virtuously, is tempted to behave wickedly, and, like the audience, learns about virtue and vice from the actions of the other characters.

The morality play moves people toward admired actions—this is the meaning of "exemplary"—and away from disparaged ones. It is a way of encoding social, professional, and moral information about someone. This information is judgmental, encompassing amusement, admiration, ridicule, and disapprobation (for example, "Dr. X's meal ticket"). I suspect a similar attribution of roles occurs not only among surgeons and other medical specialists but also among members of most comparatively stable face-to-face groupings. It involves a kind of shorthand, a summing up of socially and emotionally weighted information about a fellow member. Members are presented, described, evaluated, by being fitted into a set of culturally meaningful roles or categories. These are powerful because of their parsimony: much is left unsaid, is assumed, or is communicated on an emotional, nonrational level.

Philosopher Arthur Lovejoy analyzed seventeenth- and eighteenth-century notions of human nature, exploring the role of certain human "passions" in motivating behavior.[35] The motives or desires noted by Lovejoy include: *approbativeness,* the desire for approval or admiration of oneself, one's acts, and one's achievements on the part of one's fellows; *self esteem*, the propensity to or desire for a "good opinion" of oneself and one's qualities, acts, and achievements; and *emulativeness*, the craving for a belief in one's own superiority to others in one or another or all of these respects, and a desire for the recognition of this superiority by those with whom one associates, and for the express admission of it by them. These motives, or "springs of action,"[36] determine voluntary choices on how to behave; they are, therefore, linked to morality, to judgments of the behavior of others, and notions of how one, oneself, "ought" to behave.

It is not surprising that these desires—for approval and admiration, for self-esteem, and for a feeling of superiority—which seventeenth- and eighteenth-century writers, and apparently Lovejoy, himself, believed to be universal and dominant human "passions," motivate the behavior of surgeons.[37] Admiration, ridicule, and the attribution of roles in the surgical morality play affect modeling and self-monitoring, acting as pressures for self-regulation. Because their effect is subtle, informal, and unmentioned, these self-regulatory mechanisms have been ignored by critics, who assert that no forces for social control exist among surgeons. I suspect that surgeons themselves are not overtly aware of what is going on—although I believe they would concur if these mechanisms were pointed out to them.

Naturally, this kind of informal regulation has limitations. Those surgeons who do not care about the opinion of their fellows remain untouched by ridicule, unmoved by the desire for admiration. When one of the many hospitals where the Sleazy Surgeon (whose colleague called him "a disaster") operated on private patients wanted to review his charts, he refused to allow hospital representatives to touch them, contending that only a surgeon from a top hospital in the nearby metropolitan area was qualified to review *him*. Since he operated at suburban community hospitals, he managed to remain (or appear to be) unmoved by his colleagues' poor opinions of his behavior. Some people, then, whom one can characterize as "psychopaths," "sociopaths," or "wicked"—depending upon one's explanatory framework—are resistant to regulatory mechanisms. Such people, however, resist not only subtle informal mechanisms for social control, such as admiration, gossip, and the attribution of roles in the morality play, but also far more formal, overt, and coercive mechanisms. (Regulation of behavior is simpler in the medieval morality play, where the ultimate rewards and retribution come from God.)

I have used the terms "fellowship" and "community" to refer to a face-to-face grouping of surgeons who operate at the same hospital(s) and see each other several times a week. Because many surgeons operate at more than one hospital, the grouping is not bounded. A wider fellowship, or network, of surgeons extends across the United States. Academic surgeons who belong to prestigious surgical societies know one another; they meet at conferences, review one another's journal articles, and gossip about each others' career circumstances. Surgeons who trained together, especially at elite institutions, keep track of one another. Those who were trained by a celebrated surgeon may form a closely knit, coast-to-coast network. Chiefs of surgery know each other, about each other, and about their colleagues' hospitals and departments of surgery. If a hospital has a teaching program (with surgical house officers), the chief belongs to the Association of Program Directors in Surgery. With approximately 280 members, "it's a very tight club," said a chief, adding, "and it's getting even closer because our backs are to the wall." (When I asked why their backs were to the wall, he responded, "Because of the 'regs.' " For a discussion of the regulations affecting surgeons, see Chapter 8.)

The local fellowship of surgeons is situated within a larger fellowship of doctors, who practice at the same hospital(s). Surgeons work closely with radiologists, who x-ray and scan their patients and help interpret the results, and with pathologists, who analyze tissue specimens sent from the operating room. They share patients with "medical doctors," who are frequently responsible for the decision to send the patient to a particular surgeon, rather than to a competitor. "Lines of referral" are vital to surgeons. Certain specialists "feed" patients to certain surgeons; their goodwill is essential to a surgeon in private practice, who relies on these patients for his income. One house officer called a practice group of gastroenterologists who sent all their patients who needed colon surgery to a particular surgical group, "the goose that laid the golden egg." He said of the surgeons, "That's their bread and butter." ("Feeding" patients nourishes surgeons.) Said one man, coarser—or perhaps more honest—than his colleagues, as he dialed the number of the referring internist immediately after an operation, "Here's where I kiss ass!" He explained, "I call the referring doctor before I call the wife!" Although surgeons joke about members of other medical specialties, especially internists, they unite when threatened by outsiders.[38]

The local fellowship, or community, of doctors is placed within a larger community, where the doctors live and from which they draw their patients. In smaller communities, surgeons are known—if only by reputation. Community members have their own notions about how they want their doctors to behave and, on occasion, they are quite successful in enforcing their standards. I studied hospitals in closely knit communities where surgeons made it clear that much of their advice and many of their decisions were influenced more by community standards than by the results of the newest scientific studies. Thus, decisions, such as whether to excise a small cancerous mass (a lumpectomy) or to remove the entire breast (a mastectomy) for breast cancer, or in colon surgery, whether to give the patient a "colostomy" (passing a severed end of colon through the abdominal wall) or to hook the severed ends of bowel back together (see Chapter 6), were influenced by surgeons' interpretations of community opinion. Explaining clinical judgment, one man told me that it differs in every case and must be tempered by what people think. If you get a "talker," he said, who feels a family member has been treated badly, "that person will start talking and whole parts of the Peninsula will walk away and never come to you again!"

In summary, then, the fellowship of surgeons, within which surgeons who work in the same hospitals know about and judge one another's behavior, offers informal mechanisms for self-regulation. Gossip, jokes, and snide remarks accentuate and help enforce group standards. So does the attribution of roles in a surgical morality play, where various members embody admired and disesteemed characteristics. Within the fellowship, the desires for approval and admiration, for self-esteem, and for a feeling of superiority, motivate behavior. Without the existence of the fellowship, admiration would not lead to modeling, nor ridicule to self-monitoring, both of which result in self-regulation.

But, the fellowship has a price. The "tight group" gets even tighter when members' "backs are against the wall." When menaced by the outside world, members close ranks. This holds for almost every small community or primary group. With surgeons, closing ranks may involve joining to circumvent what members believe are foolish, dangerous, and uninformed regulations. Or, it may involve uniting to save the skin of someone recognized by colleagues as a Sleazy Surgeon. If we want surgeons to be more than "a swarm of technicians . . . with their lawyers and accountants," the fellowship is vital. The price, however, is considerable.

4

COSTING OUT MIRACLES: THE BUSINESS OF SURGERY

The typical mode of medical practice in the United States is "solo practice." This involves a man working by himself in an office which he secures and equips with his own capital, with patients who have freely chosen him as their personal physician and for whom he assumes responsibility.

Eliot Freidson
Profession of Medicine: A Study of
The Sociology of Applied Knowledge (1970)

Increasingly, the gains of one physician, or group of physicians, will have to come at the expense of other physicians or other providers. In the language of game theory, medical services in the 1980s will become more of a zero-sum game. New physicians may no longer be able to introduce an additional layer of specialized services into a community on top of what other practitioners offer. They will have to take business away from someone else.

Paul Starr
The Social Transformation of American
Medicine: The Rise of a Sovereign Profession
and the Making of a Vast Industry (1982)

Even in America, the free-standing, independent medical
practitioner has become an endangered species.

James F. Drane
Becoming a Good Doctor: The Place of
Virtue and Character in Medical Ethics (1988)

SURGERY IS not only an art, a craft, and a science; it is also
a business. Its cost is reckoned in hundreds or thousands
of dollars—whether or not the patient can afford the fee,[1]
whether or not the surgeon has achieved a cure. The business
aspects of surgery disturb many patients, who presume that
those with special powers should concern themselves with
more important matters than grubby financial details.

We are ambivalent about money in the United States.
Believing that spectacular performances—by athletes, actors,
surgeons—deserve spectacular rewards, we are, nevertheless,
offended by the affluence of those so generously rewarded.
Convinced that a surgical "miracle" is priceless, we take exception to putting a price on human lives. Respecting those
who display the signs of worldly success, we resent paying for
that success from our own finite resources.

The business of surgery exacts a cost from surgeons as well
as patients. Those who are truly unconcerned with grubby
financial details engage in the private practice of surgery at
their risk—especially today, with escalating practice costs, fees
coming under restrictive regulation, and the supply of surgeons gradually outstripping the demand for their services.
Those who are overconcerned with finances are at moral risk
—of becoming a kind of grisly entrepreneur, trafficking in
human sickness, hope, and despair.

I do not discuss the economics of medicine; it is a highly
specialized area of expertise, with its own sophisticated literature. Instead, I explore the relation of the surgeons I studied
to the business of surgery.[2]

In thirty-three months of studying surgeons (and thirty years as a doctor's wife), I encountered a variety of attitudes toward the business of medicine. "It makes me feel like a dentist!" one young physician grumbled, resisting colleagues' suggestions that he calculate the costs of running his office and bill accordingly for each minute spent with patients or, alternatively, limit the time and attention he gave. Others were able to quote to the last penny their monthly disbursements for office rent, salaries, technical equipment, and insurance, and knew just how much to bill in order to show a profit. Some read the *Wall Street Journal* and discussed investments with colleagues; others focused on patients, techniques, and concepts. I found no correlation whatsoever—negative or positive—between financial acumen and clinical ability.

I asked few direct questions about money while conducting research. These days, people are often embarrassingly frank about their sex lives, but money is a delicate subject. Surgeons would occasionally inquire about my husband's rent, secretaries' salaries, and so forth, and when I responded, might volunteer similar bits of information. Young surgeons, in their first year or two of solo practice, were more forthcoming. Naturally, they had more time to talk to me—frequently, far more time than they wished—and their confidences may have been encouraged by my evident interest in, and sympathy for, their high monthly costs and low receipts, their overwhelming medical-school debts, and their fear that, given the number and quality of competing surgeons, there were no longer enough surgical patients in their area to keep them busy.

As an anthropologist, a doctor's wife (at the time), and a middle-class American woman, I observed surgeons' private offices and added up what I saw: Was the neighborhood elegant? Was the office on "Doctors' Row"—always a high-rent location? Did the surgeon, or group, own the building? If so, did the building contain income-producing tenants? Was the office well maintained, attractively decorated, comfortably furnished? How many examining rooms did each office suite have; how many surgeons used them at the same time? (Busy doctors save time when they have enough examining rooms to contain patients in various stages of undress: removing their clothes; gowned and waiting to be examined; getting dressed again.) How many secretaries, receptionists, nurses were present during office hours? How knowledgeably did they answer the phone(s), respond to patients' questions, fulfill their employers' requests (the more highly trained, the more highly paid)? How busy were the office hours; how many patients were seen? Were patients working-class, middle-class, or well-to-do? (I won't catalog how I added up patients' clothes, jewelry, and speech, but naturally, I did.) How often did the phone ring during "hours" with calls from patients and referring doctors? Not surprisingly, I found enormous variation: in the number of patients clamoring to see a particular surgeon or group and in money spent, what that money was spent on, and what this seemed to me to show about the surgeon's attitude toward patients and money. A study of the surgical work load of the general surgeons at a medium-sized community hospital found that the busiest surgeon in the community performed more than four times as much surgery as the average; one-fourth of the surgeons did 50 percent of the work; the less busy half of the surgeons performed one-fourth of the work.[3] My observations confirmed this disparity.

THREE SURGEONS IN PRIVATE PRACTICE

To explore the range of attitudes and behavior regarding the business of surgery, let us observe three private practitioners. First, we will visit the office of Dr. Santora, a semiretired orthopedist in his sixties, who sees patients but no longer operates. He has two partners—one of whom is his son—and three (what he and his partners call) "girls" working for him.

An Exemplary Surgeon

The Santora group rents space in a large, rather plain building, conveniently located in a shopping center near Reid General Hospital. Santora's brother, who is an internist, has an office next door, which he shares with Santora's daughter, who is also an internist. Although they had one of the largest offices for the private practice of surgery I've ever seen, the Santora surgical group was about to take over more space. Before expanding, the office contained: three examining rooms (they will have five); three consulting rooms (where the doctor talks with patients before or after examining them); an X-ray room; and an air-conditioned computer room, containing an unusually large computer, microfilmed medical records dating from 1948, when Santora began to practice, and a microfilm reader. Santora told me that the group subscribes to a library service that enables them to retrieve journal articles via computer, and that the partners can telephone from the hospital to insert or retrieve information from the computer. They also possess a device that makes Polaroid transparencies from X rays, so that the films can be mailed or used for lectures. Every consulting and examining room contains a special telephone for dictating letters and notes. Before dictating, the partners press a button to select one of four different "tanks," or reels; a letter dictated on reel number one will be ready in a few minutes; case studies are dictated on another reel. Their "girls" turn these into letters for insurance examinations. The surgeons also send letters to referring doctors, outlining their findings.

Santora said that their "girls" have been with them "forever"; he asked one woman how long she had worked for him and she responded, "Twenty years." Their one new employee had been Santora's patient when she was a child. He told me that they have profit sharing for the "girls," which really motivates them when they collect fees.

Field Notes. It's the best-run office I've ever seen. . . . Santora said several times that he doesn't want to get rich and doesn't want partners who want to. They do a lot of their work by telephone. It takes two months to get an appointment, and they encourage a lot of their patients to telephone in and report their progress. They dictate notes on the telephone calls as well as the office visits; he [Santora] likes to do this dictation [notes on the office visits] in front of the patient; it gets done, and if he makes a little mistake, the patient corrects him.

He saw a patient with a swollen finger—used to be called a "baseball finger," he said. She comes in every ten days or so, and they put a new splint on it. They'd get more money if they operated, he said, but this is a better way—less deforming, less expensive.

He saw a young man who had hurt his shoulder playing football. . . . He showed [his chart] to me, pointing out how many orthopedic problems the kid had had throughout his life. Some people just do. He wonders why; they're all real problems, too. It's not a very happy family. . . . After seeing the boy, he said to me, "He seems happy, but he bites his nails so deeply, and he isn't settled in school." . . . He thinks he's not happy. . . . He wishes he had more time, he said, to find out more about persons; that's not supposed to be a doctor's job, but he thinks it's important to touch people and heal them and know about them as persons.

He looks at the patient first, and *then* at the X ray, so he doesn't get preconceptions from the X ray; that's called "riding the X ray." . . . He sees patients in his consulting room first, then puts them in the examining room. Freddy and Jack [his partners] put them in the examining room first, he said. He sees fewer patients this way, but he likes it better. He doesn't want to stack up patients and have too many put in so he has to rush each patient. "I don't want to get rich," he said, again.

Actually, he took time with each patient; as Jack Viera [his partner] said, he *teaches* each of them, tells what is wrong, what he will do, what they can do to help it. Rather than being *nice* the way Hardy is [another surgeon whose office hours I had observed a few days earlier] or charming, he's direct, talks to them as he would talk to anyone, not up, not down, but carefully, making sure they understand.

All the babies and little kids seemed to go for him directly—

the babies smiled at him, grabbed his hand, etc., although he didn't seem to cluck or "goo-goo" at them. Mentioned, though, that his wife and he had taken one baby for three months. She needed special treatment . . . and the mother asked if they would keep her. He'd go home every lunch hour to play with the baby, and the kids [his son and daughter], who were young then, just loved her, as did his wife. He said a few times, of a particularly cute baby, "I'll take that one," and I think he really *meant* it.

Dr. Santora is a remarkable surgeon—a remarkable human being (which is why I am choosing to present an orthopedist, rather than the general surgeons my research concentrated on). He is known, respected, and beloved in the area. I believed Santora when he said he did not want to get rich; if he had wanted to he would not have invested in all that expensive technology, which makes the practice more *efficient* but probably impresses patients far less than a fancy building or luxurious, as opposed to comfortable, furnishings.

Santora may not want to get rich, but he's a good businessman.[4] He keeps in close touch with referring doctors, which stimulates further referrals; he has profit sharing, to encourage efficient fee collection. Santora told how he had been active in community service and medical politics when he was younger—excellent ways for a young doctor to catch the attention of potential patients and referring doctors. His son has continued the tradition; at the time of my fieldwork, Freddy was president of the local medical society. (In addition, I heard gossip that Santora had used his influence to limit the number of competing orthopedists given operating privileges at Reid General Hospital.)

A Sleazy Surgeon

Now, let us observe a very different kind of surgeon. Dr. Auerbach, a general surgeon in his thirties, who had "gone out on his own" the previous year and was in the process of furnishing a new office. Rumor had it that Auerbach paid "kickbacks" to nursing-home personnel who sent him patients.

Field Notes. He's a tall, slender young man, who was dressed in an extremely elegant, well-fitting suit. . . . He graduated from the University of Paris. . . . It's not so hard to survive [he told me]; he does one or two operations a week, which is enough to survive.

He borrowed fifty thousand dollars to furnish his office—he thinks it's important to do things right. . . . He has a friend who is an antiques dealer who helped him get an eighteenth-century desk, which he refinished, and some Queen Anne chairs. He thinks antiques make people feel at home and [make] the young surgeon seem trustworthy and solid.

Now, a lot of what he does is "public relations," he said. He spends a lot of time hanging around the hospital. "What do you do?" I asked. "I spend a lot of time in the cafeteria having coffee," he said. (He bought me coffee.) For example, he gave really nice-looking jars of hard candy [to the doctors and to the nurses' stations] for Christmas. They were so attractive, I noticed them. He went to [the nearby city] to get them; he wants them to be remembered. If he gets even one patient from that, it's worthwhile.

Patients come from referrals from other doctors till you're established and patients send others [he said], and eventually you have your own patients. It's hard because people like the Vesperi group [the most successful general surgery group at Reid General Hospital] have their own patients who are not referred by others, and then they can refer their patients to internists, who reciprocate by referring patients to them. He and another surgeon are going into a weight-loss business at a nearby spa; he thinks that will help people get to know him and remember him. . . . I asked about his suit, if that was part of his image; and he said he likes to dress well; Americans don't know how to dress, but he learned in Europe; Americans dress in "polyester plastic."

He said he likes to do things his own way, not the way other people do things; that includes the way he operates. He wanted to be a plastic surgeon for a while. . . . He still likes to operate with very little openings if he can. He took me upstairs to see "his gallbladder"—the first time [at Reid General] I heard a patient referred to as a body part. The "gallbladder," a well-built, tanned young man, was as proud of the tiny scar as he [Auerbach] was.

Then, when I asked if I could see it, he took me to see his office.

> *Field Notes.* It is really *extremely* attractive; everything very new (including the old things), arranged with great taste—and expense. I got the feeling that for Dr. Auerbach, this facade is the most important element in being a successful surgeon, which to him (this is just a guess) is what being a *good* surgeon consists of.

Later, when I told the assistant director of surgery that I had seen Auerbach's office and that it was extremely attractive, he responded that it was a pity Auerbach was a bad doctor. The assistant director's summation of the young surgeon was: "Unfortunately, he has more woof than warp!"

Let us follow Auerbach, some months later, as he makes rounds upon hospitalized patients:

> *Field Notes.* We saw a lot of patients, fourteen in all. Many of them are "consults," listed as the internist's patient. He prefers that, he said. After all, that's the way surgeons really work; that way, it's the internist's patient, and he [Auerbach] operates when and if necessary. (Since he gets paid by the operation, it means the internist does the care.)
>
> We stopped to see an old black lady from a nursing home; he had done a debridement [removing foreign matter and tissue from a wound] at the bedside yesterday, he said. When I said, "Don't you need a sterile OR for that?" he said, "No, it was dead skin; she felt no pain." As we got there, the patient was being examined by a small group, and her IV [intravenous] tube, fixed in the side of her face near the neck, popped out. "Just in time," said one young man. "Sure," said Auerbach, and with great patience and good temper started trying to get another IV in. He kept poking with a great big needle into the patient's face, she kept moaning, and he kept missing. One young man—a male nurse, I think—kept wincing and patting the patient and saying there, there, Annie. . . . But Auerbach didn't turn a hair; he kept on

poking her again and again with that giant needle as though she were an animal—no, not an animal, a plant or something that felt *no* pain. Finally, he got it in and they put the IV in, but the liquid squirted out through some of the holes that had been made. He ended up making a "temporary" attachment in her hand as she moaned (she did not seem with it, but she *did* moan quite loudly every time he poked her with the needle) and promising to come back later to do a permanent one. A very pretty young woman was helping him and flirting with him. She wanted to see him do a "cutdown," which is what he would have to do for the next IV; he said he'd call her. . . . (I had the feeling there might be something between the two of them; he said she was a third-year medical resident.)

[He told me about his surgical training and described the man who trained him, whose investments have made him a millionaire.] I bet he'll end up a millionaire, I said (I bet he will!), pleasing him. "I need lots of money," he said.

He examined an ulcer on the foot of another old man, and squeezed it hard to see how it was doing. The old man was another zonked nursing-home patient, but it obviously hurt a lot. Auerbach didn't wince; it didn't seem to affect him in the slightest.

I asked him if caring was important. No, he said. What matters more than the surgeon caring is the patient's state of mind. The patient has to *want* to get better; some people just give up. What's important between patient and surgeon is "a lot of public relations. That's the art," he said. "That's what affects how successful you'll be."

Later that day, when I asked him how he happened to become a doctor, he laughed and replied: "Money," adding, with more gravity, "No. I always liked it and wanted to do it since I was a kid."

These comparisons are, admittedly, extreme. One surgeon is nearing the end of an honorable—and honored—career; the other is at the beginning of what promises to be a lucrative career. One is successful, and the other probably will be—but each defines success very differently. Both are good business-

men, although the business of surgery is apparently secondary to one and primary to the other.

Both Santora and Auerbach practice at Reid General Hospital, a well-run, well-endowed, medium-sized suburban community hospital in a tightly knit community. The Santora family (two brothers who practice surgery and medicine at the hospital with two members of the younger generation also practicing surgery and medicine there) was one of four such medical dynasties there. Santora's son, Freddy, and Auerbach both received their surgical training at Reid General.

A Foreign Medical Graduate (FMG)

Now, let us observe an entirely different kind of practice, based in a very different kind of hospital. I shall call this medium-sized urban hospital with a less than stellar reputation "Mount Saint Elsewhere," which is "the general designation for the lower class of hospitals . . . definitely derogatory."[5] When I visited its new chief of surgery to request permission to study his department, he inquired why I wanted to study self-regulation among surgeons, asserting that, from what he's seen of the surgeons in that area, there is *no* self-regulation. "I don't want to be chauvinistic," he said, "but let's put it this way: different cultures seem to have different standards about lying. I've had surgeons from other cultures look me straight in the eye and lie. I knew they were lying," he said, "and they knew I knew. But still they lied. They just have different standards of morality!" declared the chief. (The chief was suggesting that the foreign-born and foreign-educated surgeons in that area had lower standards, in surgery as well as morality, than those of native-born and native-educated surgeons—such as himself.)

The chief did not allow me to study his hospital; he did, however, find a surgeon willing to let me observe him for several weeks. If Dr. Moslevi lied, he was skillful enough to conceal it from me. Moslevi, an affable, chunky, sallow-skinned man, who graduated from medical school in Teheran and was trained as a surgeon at Mount Saint Elsewhere, had exquisite manners: he opened doors, tendered chairs, held coats for me, his office staff, and his female patients. First, let's observe him as he makes rounds on his patients, and those of his partner, Dr. Singh:

> *Field Notes.* We saw six patients in the hospital. Usually they have between ten and twenty, but it's a slow time, he said. Most seemed to be working-class or lower-middle-class; ditto for his office patients, later. He said High Point [an upper-middle-class neighborhood near the hospital] does not really support Mount Saint Elsewhere. . . . He also has an office in Southside [an ethnic neighborhood], where he lives, and he occasionally uses Southside Hospital [a small proprietary hospital with a poor reputation].
>
> He made a "consult" on an old man who had a hip operation who seemed to be obstructed. . . . After X rays and a barium enema, which showed that he [the patient] was blocked from an incarcerated hernia, Moslevi decided he had to operate. Then it was a question of getting an operating room; they are very inefficient at Mount Saint Elsewhere, he said, unless the patient is bleeding to death. The final decision was that the operation would take place that evening.
>
> He [then] had to go to "utilization review" [a hospital committee that reviews the stays of hospitalized patients] to justify the hospital stay of a patient workmen's compensation had just disallowed. But they [workmen's compensation processors] had authorized that operation, he said. "They're counting on the fact that two years later, the clerk will have lost the authorization," he said. "But I have a copy!" I said that didn't seem very fair, and he said, "Yes, they fight dirty." For example, they'll correspond with you about a current patient for six months but neglect to tell you that the patient isn't covered by them for one reason or another; they'll tell you after the whole thing is over.
>
> After rounds, he went to "clean up" his charts; he had to dic-

tate ten charts.[6] . . . In the dictation was a colon resection, and I noted the anastomosis [joining] was done by hand; I mentioned this to him afterwards, and he said, yes, after all he has a responsibility to teach house officers. Besides, . . . sometimes it [the special stapler] isn't available; the hospital is eighteen months behind in its payments to vendors, and sometimes they don't have the equipment. . . . He said the people in charge of getting supplies work about an hour a day and then spend about seven hours a day drinking coffee and looking at new equipment, and sometimes they just don't get around to replacing equipment that's needed.

Through the day, Moslevi kept coming back to the theme of how badly the hospital was run. He said that in the old days, nurses nursed instead of spending all of their time at meetings. Twenty years ago, one nurse used to run the OR; she would sit outside the operating rooms from 7:00 A.M. to 5:00 P.M. making sure everything ran well. She had two assistants, and everything ran perfectly. Now, they have twenty-five people, and everything runs abysmally. They fired all the nurses who did not have B.A.'s, he said, but the ones who do are just passing through on their way to graduate school. If you hold out your hand during an operation, the nurses don't know what to put in it; if you ask for the instrument by name, they don't even know the names. There's no one there to take care of the patients, he complained; he'd just like someone, *anyone,* to be able to feed the old sick patients, that person doesn't need a fancy degree. But the hospital has many more secretaries than nurses, and the nurses don't nurse, and the supervisors never go to the floors, so things run very badly, he concluded.

Dr. Moslevi has an office in a large, somewhat drab medical building not far from the hospital. He apologized for the condition of his office, telling me that they were in the middle of redecorating. He was using a painter whose notice he had seen around the neighborhood, a part-time teacher who took on odd painting jobs. Because the man worked irregular hours, it had taken more than two weeks to finish painting. The office was small, with two tiny examining rooms, a cramped waiting room, Moslevi's consulting room, and a room containing three female employees. Each room opened onto the next; in some, it was necessary to move a chair to open the door to the adjoining room. Although I had been studying surgeons for almost a year and a half, Moslevi's practice, his office, and his way of doing things, were new to me.

> *Field Notes.* From 1:30 to about 6:15, he saw thirteen patients (which is not all that many compared to the surgeons I watched [previously]). They came in two waves, one at the beginning, then a lull, the second after 5:00 P.M., when people get out of work. Of these thirteen, I would estimate that three were middle-class.
>
> I find the office really depressing, and I don't think it's just that it's still being painted. He's been there ten years, but it all looks as though he bought everything secondhand ten years ago. The secretary's typewriter is an old Underwood, not electric. This office is much plainer [than the surgeons' offices I had previously observed]. The newly painted peach and magenta color scheme is claustrophobic; his private consultation room has no windows (the secretaries have the room with a window); the new carpeting has a kind of ghastly pattern on it. . . . I think it may be social class—not necessarily his [Moslevi's], but the kind of practice he runs. Surely lots of the Reid General doctors have working-class patients, but somehow they run a different kind of operation. [There is] some attempt, mainly successful, to look classy, and run it in a classy way. . . . He talks nicely to patients, the same way he talks to me. [He] doesn't seem to change his manner for different genders or different social classes. He's just a *nice* man, or seems to be.

During a hiatus between the two waves of patients, Moslevi told me that, during his first year of practice, the office building went on the market for $200,000 in cash. He tried to organize ten doctors to put in $20,000 each, or twenty doctors to put $10,000 each, but his colleagues kept dragging their feet, saying they needed to inspect the electricity and the furnace. As they waited for the furnace to be examined, the building was sold. Two years later, the building was sold again, for $2.5 million dollars; a few years later, it went again, for $4 million. The new owners co-oped the building and made $6 million dollars on the deal, he said. Moslevi told me that he now owns his office, and only now that the building is co-oped is it finally getting a new furnace and electricity—which must be paid for by the doctors who own the offices.

The thirteen patients Moslevi saw that day included a predominance of Iranians, some of whom spoke no English, several working-class Italians, and three apparently middle-class people recovering from accidents and injuries (who I speculated might have come to him via the emergency room of Mount Saint Elsewhere). In my field notes I wondered whether the fancy office was an American invention, or at least whether the absolute need for one was an American cultural need.

My experiences with Mount Saint Elsewhere and Dr. Moslevi point to a gap in my data: I have little information about "the lower class of hospitals"[7] and the primarily foreign-born and foreign-educated surgeons who staff them.[8] The networks through which I secured surgeons originated with my former husband, who attended an elite American medical school and practices at a university hospital attached to another major medical school and university. These networks extended *out*, but not that far *down*. Although one of the four hospitals I studied in depth was a public hospital located in an urban ghetto, it was a university hospital associated with a medical school; none of the hospitals I concentrated on could be described disparagingly as "Mount Saint Elsewhere." My former husband, who started working in hospitals at the age of fifteen, said he could identify a good hospital the moment he entered the front door—by the smell. At Mount Saint Elsewhere, I learned what he meant. Wherever one went in Reid

General Hospital—lobbies, public hallways, wards, dressing rooms, bathrooms—one encountered attendants busily mopping and cleaning; a clean, antiseptic scent permeated the hospital. I assumed this was the way hospitals smelled—until Mount Saint Elsewhere. Mount Saint Elsewhere did *not* smell clean. When I went to the ladies' room, it was dirty. The burly armed guards at Reid General were intimidatingly serious: whenever I climbed the back stairs or ventured anywhere outside the public spaces, I was firmly questioned by a guard, who would match my face to the photo on my plastic identification card before letting me pass. At Mount Saint Elsewhere, I entered the doctor's entrance daily, with no identification card (by this time, I knew how to find shortcuts, even in strange hospitals); the guards were so busy talking to one another that they ignored me. No one seemed to notice or care where I went. I even penetrated the operating-room suite without identification or permission.[9] Dr. Moslevi's complaints about the hospital's lack of equipment and nurses had a certain ritual quality—many surgeons grouse about a shortage of personnel and supplies; but, although they may have been exaggerated, Moslevi's remarks had an edge of seriousness that similar complaints lack. I believe Mount Saint Elsewhere *was* badly run, and in serious financial difficulties.

Moslevi is the graduate of a foreign medical school (an FMG); he was trained at a nonelite program; he practices at a badly run, low-prestige hospital. I cannot evaluate his surgical skills; I was not allowed to study his hospital or observe operations there. He is an amiable and considerate man, and his politeness extended to me, his patients, and his staff; he seemed honest and concerned about his patients; and I suspect that if he had had too much to hide, he would not have volunteered to let me follow him for several weeks.

But, unlike Dr. Santora, whose patients must wait two months for an appointment, or Dr. Auerbach, who "needs lots of money" and seems well on the way to obtaining it,[10]

Moslevi does not appear to be particularly busy or success-ful. His office hours are not crowded; he and Dr. Singh have relatively few hospitalized patients; and he makes leisurely rounds, taking several hours to finish tasks that busier doctors accomplish in twenty minutes. Moslevi scrambles for patients. He sees many Iranians, from a wide geographic area; he runs a biweekly surgical clinic for a cafeteria worker's union, from which he gets patients; he operates on workmen's compensa-tion cases (avoided by busier surgeons, because of difficulties in reimbursement); he obtains patients from the Mount Saint Elsewhere emergency room (who return to their elite doc-tors after being treated for the condition that brought them to the ER). But Moslevi does not have to be particularly busy in order to make a decent, if not luxurious, living.[11] Surgical fees are steep; whatever the social class of the patient, the fees are frequently paid by a "third party"—a union health plan, work-men's compensation, Medicare, Medicaid, or private medical insurance.

Despite his scarcity of patients, Moslevi appears to have business acumen. His income may be relatively low compared to that of busier surgeons, but then, he is cautious about ex-penses. Although he economizes on office decoration—and it is conceivable that an office that seemed shabby and depress-ing to me makes his foreign-born patients feel very much at home—he has three employees. Moreover, only the caution of his colleagues and his own lack of funds prevented him from buying his office building, which would have made good business sense.

Business sense is critical for a private practitioner. Office rent is high for appropriate locations that can be reached easily by patients. Salaries for trained technicians, receptionists, and secretaries can also be substantial—and untrained ones may be inefficient in scheduling patients, keeping records, and bill-ing for services. A shabby office, with careless, rude, or slow-witted personnel says something about the doctor: his competence, judgment, success. Patients, as the young surgeon noted when discussing a surgeon's looks, are very perceptive, and the appearance of the office and the behavior of employees can also help inspire trust—or distrust. An attractive office is helpful—especially for a young doctor, with little reputation and few patients. Looking successful, as Dr. Auerbach knew, can lead to success in the business of surgery. Doctors must, however, have some sense of how to balance outgo against income; if they spend too much and earn too little, they're going to get into financial difficulties. Being in the private practice of medicine (as a doctor I knew used to say) is in some ways like running a candy store or other small retail business: someone has to always be there "minding the store."[12] Money comes in *only* when the practitioner is working, while money is flowing out continuously on rent, salaries, technical equipment, and insurance. Moreover, self-employed doctors must arrange for their retirement; the income lasts only as long as they are practicing. This is all rather basic, even simple-minded. But many young doctors learn these simple financial facts the hard way; medical schools give no instruction on the business of medicine, and a talent for medicine does not guarantee a similar talent for business.

Let me repeat that a talent for business does *not* indicate that a doctor lacks a talent for medicine. The real question is which comes first, business or medicine. For some surgeons I observed, medicine seemed to come in a poor second to money. And, venality is a deadly surgical sin—perhaps the deadliest (see Chapter 7).

AN EXEMPLARY SURGEON IN A PREPAID HEALTH PLAN

When money comes in *too* poor a second to surgery, however, the surgeon may do well to avoid private practice. I encoun-

tered one such surgeon, who worked on a salaried basis for
one type of prepaid health plan, a health maintenance organization (HMO). Although the health plan had low prestige
at his hospital, Dr. Lan was characterized by colleagues as an
"A-plus surgeon." He told me that prepaid care may be "the
future of medicine," and after seeing Lan operate and talk with
patients, the future did not seem all that bleak.[13] When examining patients, he did something I've never seen anyone
else do: before putting his stethoscope to bare flesh, he quietly
warmed it in his palm. Lan explained why so many patients
were scheduled for breast examinations the day I observed his
office hours: he encourages women with fibrocystic disease
(who develop frequent breast cysts, which, although usually
benign, can be worrisome) to see him every three months for
a checkup. "After all, it's prepaid," he tells them, "Why not
take advantage of it? Instead of being sure every year, the way
they do 'outside,' you can be sure every three months." Dr. Lan
mentioned the way things were done "outside" several times;
he seemed far more comfortable "inside." One elderly lady,
whom he characterized as a difficult patient, came to see him
just to talk. He said she sometimes talks for half an hour. "It's
irrelevant to the matter at hand," he reported, "but I feel she
needs the opportunity to air herself out, so I listen."[14] When
a health-plan administrator came to his office to discuss bill-
ing, Lan told her to take whatever Medicaid offered for one
patient and not bill for the remainder, because the patient had
no money. "I can afford to do this because I'm paid a salary
by [the group], while perhaps other surgeons can't because
they have to pay their overhead," he explained. Later, when he
told the administrator to forget another bill, he shrugged his
shoulders, and said ruefully, "I'd never survive outside!" (The
patients whose bills he canceled were his own private, fee-
for-service patients; the doctors were permitted to see private
patients at the HMO offices.)

Many surgeons expressed fears that prepaid national health

care might be the future of medicine, but only one, a resident trained in Great Britain, spoke approvingly of this possible "future." Isaak, who came to the United States because there were so few positions for surgeons in Britain, was convinced that patients were given better care, and doctors more respect, in Great Britain. Surgery is a business in the United States, he stated; in Britain, it's an art (he was convinced that art and business were antithetical). In the United States, everything is regulated, he complained—drugs, licenses, training, everything—and everyone sues doctors, yet none of the regulations or lawsuits make doctors honest; he still sees patients operated on who probably should not be. In Europe, on the other hand, no regulation exists, but the doctors regulate themselves, said Isaak.

Dr. Lan was not the only salaried surgeon I met who seemed to be relatively disinterested in money. I encountered a number of salaried academic surgeons who seemed far more involved in their work than in augmenting what they described as perfectly adequate salaries. Being salaried, however, did not automatically guarantee a lack of business aptitude or disinterest in money.

"FULL-TIME" MEN

Among the salaried surgeons I observed were "full-time" academic surgeons at university hospitals associated with medical schools. At one such hospital, a chief of surgery told me that there is an unwritten formula that calculates how much lower than the income of a private practitioner an academic salary can be without losing the doctor. "Harvard or Yale can pay 30 percent to 40 percent less; a medical college with a lesser reputation must pay 10 percent to 15 percent less," he said. He said that his school allows surgeons to keep the money they make operating on their own private patients—after a certain share is apportioned to the dean of the medical school and the department of surgery. Consequently, surgeons can approximate the earnings of an average surgeon in their community.[15]

A number of academic surgeons told me how they are not as interested in money as "some doctors"; their self-righteous tone of voice implied that, unlike practitioners, *they* cared only for the art, craft, and science of surgery. However, in one academic department where several "full-time" men repeatedly mentioned how much less they earned than their practitioner friends, I was surprised to learn from a young surgeon who had finished his residency a year and a half before, that he had earned ninety-four thousand dollars the previous year[16]—plus "incentives" for patient care.[17] Fees seemed to play a significant role in the prestige ranking system among these academic surgeons; the men who brought in money for the department acted somewhat superior to those who did not. *"We* pay our way," said the chief proudly, about his department. Everyone in this department seemed to be interested in and aware of just how much extra money his colleagues were earning from various outside sources, such as patient incentives and testing products for drug companies.

Despite the financial complaints of some full-time men, those surgeons who were really hungry were young practitioners who were employed by established groups and hoping to become a partner, or who had recently "gone out on their own."[18] At Reid General Hospital, an older surgeon predicted that the young surgeons there will perform half the number of operations he and his partners do and earn a quarter of their incomes. "They're not gonna make the megabucks," he asserted.[19]

When I submitted a paper on surgeons to a British journal, the editor requested some background information, suggesting that I explain, for example, that in the United States, surgeons are "rich white men." I did indeed observe a large number of rich white—as well as rich Asian and Oriental—

men practicing surgery, but I also observed a growing number of white, Asian, and Oriental men (and a few women) who were desperately worried about their professional and financial futures.[20] These were people who had spent ten years— sometimes longer—training to become doctors and then surgeons. Many were devoted to their patients and to the art, craft, and science of surgery. For every Dr. Auerbach, I met a number of honest and accomplished young surgeons, caught between rigorous and expensive training requirements, and reimbursement patterns and patient availability that were shrinking so rapidly that one might wonder whether only somewhat sleazy surgeons could make a success of the solo practice of surgery.[21]

Perhaps success in practice is determined by more than either the "sleaze factor" or American birth and education. Older colleagues, who characterized a number of the hungriest young surgeons as "not aggressive enough," could not, or would not, explain exactly what they meant by "aggressive." I noticed, however, that the young surgeons who had the highest profiles and evinced the most confidence were those most likely to be invited to join the most active practice groups— and to have more patients when they went out into practice on their own. An internist once characterized certain practitioners as "patient-prone." To return to what the extremely successful surgeon said about confidence: "You've got to seduce the patient, you've got to convince them that you're the best possible surgeon, that you've got everything under control, that they're going to get better fast. You've got to seduce the referring doctor, convince him you're the best possible person to send the case to. You've got to seduce the family, and make them feel confidence in you." It is conceivable that the confidence necessary to carry off surgical "miracles" is equally effective in achieving success in private practice. What we cannot know is how long the private practice of surgery will remain a business, and if it does not remain one, what will replace it. The future of surgery is unclear. Perhaps it will be salaried practice, with surgeons working for health maintenance organizations, a national health plan, or for-profit hospitals.[22] Or, perhaps the future will mirror and magnify the present, with an ever-increasing number of surgeons hungrily competing for a static pool of patients. If so, young surgeons will pay a high price, in blasted hopes and crushing debts—or in a growing pressure to engage in somewhat sleazy practices—in order to enter and attempt to succeed in the business of surgery.

5

A DAY WITH A COMPASSIONATE YOUNG SURGEON

> Now tell, is the doctor in the precise sense, of whom you recently spoke, a money-maker or one who cares for the sick? Speak about the man who is really a doctor.
>
> Plato
> *Republic*

To become a good doctor, one must both know the truth and do the truth.

James F. Drane
Becoming a Good Doctor: The Place of
Virtue and Character in Medical Ethics

THE DAY

*D*R. BRYNA is a compassionate surgeon," said the chief resident. After ten months of observing surgeons at work, I was still struck by their martial, heroic approach to patients and illness. "Isn't that a contradiction in terms?" I inquired. "No," replied the resident, "he's unusual. If there's an old man who lives alone who needs stitches removed, Bryna would just as soon go to his home to remove the stitches; he'll visit patients at home. If a patient dies, there he is right in front at the funeral, feeling bad. He's a good surgeon," he added, "although he gets excited. If a patient bleeds or something happens, he gets tense. He's not a block of ice like his partner."

On leaving the hospital that evening, I told Dr. Bryna I was sorry I had missed the breast biopsy he had performed at 1:00 that afternoon; the operation I was observing had run into complications and lasted from 11:00 A.M. until almost 4:00. "Oh," he said, with what sounded like real emotion, "it was good news!" I did not remember hearing a surgeon speak with such intensely personal feeling about a patient's prognosis.

Some weeks later, I observed Bryna doing something else that struck me as unusual. He was operating on a black woman with high blood pressure, diabetes, and a failing kidney, who had been given local anesthesia and was consequently awake during the operation. Rather than assuming a first-name basis with the patient as did most of the surgeons, nurses, and anesthesiologists I had observed in the operating room, Bryna called the patient "Miss Washington." Although the procedure was relatively simple—inserting a new Goretex [synthetic blood vessel] graft used for kidney dialysis—it was slow, picky work, and after two and a half hours, the woman, who had been lying on her back, started groaning, complaining that her back hurt, and moving about. The more she moved, the longer the procedure took. Bryna asked the anesthesiologist to give the patient something to keep her quiet, but the anesthesiologist (a new woman, relieving the regular anesthesiologist, who had left the room for a lunch break), was busy putting cold compresses on the patient's forehead and did not respond. Bryna's composure seemed ruffled, but he did not lose his temper as I had seen some surgeons do in similar situations. He worked away, between the wriggles; spoke sternly, telling the patient to lie still, it would be over soon; and continued to address her as "Miss Washington."

Several months later, I spent a day with Dr. Bryna. We had arranged to meet at 8:00 A.M. at Rice Community Hospital, where I had been studying surgeons for more than a year. At

8:30, I received a message that Bryna's operation, scheduled for 9:30 at the neighboring Saint Augustus Medical Center, had been moved ahead to 8:30, and that I should meet him in the Saint Augustus Medical Center lobby at 10:00. (Bryna and his senior partner, Dr. Hamilton, operated at both Rice Community Hospital and Saint Augustus.) When I arrived at Saint Augustus, the lobby was empty. At 10:15, I telephoned the operating-room suite and was told that Bryna was still operating. At 10:45, a nurse phoned me in the lobby with a message that I should meet him upstairs, in the recovery room. There, he was seated in a glassed-in cubicle dictating notes about the operation he had just completed. His notes were extremely detailed, recording the kind of incision, its exact location, the kind of stitches taken, and the kind of thread.

Bryna introduced me to the patient, who was in a bed outside the dictating cubicle, with intravenous fluid running from an upended bottle into a needle in his forearm. He explained that the patient, Dr. Thomas, had been a dentist before retiring. The patient was awake but seemed slightly disoriented. "I'll see you later, when you're settled in your room," Bryna promised.

When we left the bedside, Bryna told me that he and his partner had lost three patients that week. It was "tragic," he said and appeared to mean it. ("Tragic" seemed a rare term for a surgeon to apply to the death of a patient; surgeons are so surrounded by tragedy that many appear to buffer out the sorrow and fear that permeates their contacts with patients and their families.) One of the patients they had lost was a doctor's father. Weird things always happen to doctors' families, he explained, and after all sorts of unusual complications, the man had "coded" during a procedure. "How old was he?" I asked. "Seventy-two," he responded. (Not everyone would classify the death of a seventy-two-year-old as a "tragedy," but Bryna clearly did so.) As we conversed in the recovery room, a voice kept repeating his name on the overhead loudspeaker:

"Dr. Bryna, call 8564," "Dr. Bryna, call 6321." Bryna took his time on each telephone call; he clearly enjoyed chatting and was less abrupt on the phone than most surgeons I observed.

One call came from an internist who wanted Bryna to examine a patient, who would meet him in the emergency room. The patient arrived at 11:20 accompanied by her husband. Mrs. Gordon was a pretty, delicate-looking woman of sixty-four. The husband, a retired veterinarian, withdrew to the waiting room, while Bryna examined her. Mrs. Gordon's abdomen was enormously distended; she was "obstructed," said Bryna quietly to me. "How long have you been losing weight?" he asked. (She had not said she had lost weight.) "Oh, I haven't been eating well since I had this trouble at Passover," she responded, relating how she had become nauseated at her daughter's home in Denver, where they had gone for the Passover meal. She had vomited and felt ill but did not want to hurt her daughter's feelings, so she had said little about it. The Gordons planned to spend spring vacation in Hawaii with their son, a teacher, she reported, worrying that this incident might interfere with their trip.

After examining Mrs. Gordon and looking at her X rays, which the Gordons had brought from the internist, Bryna ordered a barium enema. Out of earshot of the patient, he telephoned the operating room and asked the head nurse to set aside some time for a possible emergency operation.

We went to the waiting room to talk with the husband, a good-looking man, who appeared to be in his late sixties. Bryna gently asked the husband to sit down before discussing his wife's disorder with him. He explained that if Mrs. Gordon were obstructed, she would need an operation immediately, since she looked extremely obstructed. If she were completely obstructed, which the barium enema would show, the cecum might "blow"—or rupture—sending feces into the peritoneum, which could cause peritonitis. "Have you done many operations like this?" asked Dr. Gordon, in a doubting tone. (Bryna was thirty-four and looked younger.) "Yes, lots," responded Bryna. "Could we possibly get a second opinion?" requested the husband. "Sure," said Bryna, "is there anyone you want?" No, responded the husband, he just wanted to be able to tell people who asked that he had done everything that could possibly be done.

Bryna and I returned to the emergency room to telephone and find out who on the surgical staff was available to examine the patient and give an opinion of what was wrong and what should be done about it. "I can't get my partner; that would be unethical," he explained. It seemed to me that Bryna would have welcomed the opinion of his skilled and highly respected senior partner.

Bryna also telephoned the radiology department and discussed the barium enema. He arranged the scheduling on a very personal basis, requesting the radiology residents he wanted, by name, and asking that the procedure be done immediately, as a favor to him. We walked through the mazelike hospital corridors to radiology to oversee the barium enema. Bryna entered the room, where Mrs. Gordon had been placed on a large metal table, to reassure her that everything was proceeding as it was meant to. We then waited in the hallway as the barium was administered and the X rays taken. When the residents appeared to be having difficulties, Bryna arranged for a senior radiologist to enter the room and help them.

The minute the X-ray films emerged from the developer, Bryna carefully examined them and then brought them to the chief of radiology to confer about the findings. The chief radiologist, Bryna, and the radiology residents who examined the films all agreed: Mrs. Gordon had an "apple-core" obstruction of the large bowel. Bryna pointed it out to me on the film: in the intestine was a form shaped like the concave core of an eaten apple. The obstruction might be caused by diverticulitis, said Bryna, or by adhesions from an earlier appendectomy, but it was probably "CA" [cancer]. Bryna called the operating room a second time and asked how soon he could have a room for an emergency operation. He also telephoned Mrs. Gordon's internist to discuss the findings.

We went downstairs to the waiting room to tell Dr. Gordon that his wife needed to be operated on immediately. Perhaps an internist should give a second opinion on whether Mrs. Gordon needed an operation, said the husband. Mentioning his wife's recent loss of appetite, he remarked in a loving tone, "She's a creature who never was regular in her eating," as though Mrs. Gordon were somehow more ethereal than solid flesh-and-blood types, like himself.

After talking to their internist, the husband decided he would like a second opinion from Dr. Hamilton, Bryna's senior partner. Down came Hamilton, summoned from the operating-room suite, still dressed in "greens," tall, handsome, with an air of quiet authority. Hamilton examined Mrs. Gordon, looked at the barium-enema films, and then talked with the Gordons while Bryna and I waited outside the little emergency-room cubicle. We later learned that, when he confirmed that Mrs. Gordon needed an emergency operation, the couple had asked whether Hamilton could perform it; he told them he had operations scheduled for the entire day and could not. Said Bryna, to me, "If I had taken her [operated on her] without that [the consult], he'd [the husband] have gone wild!" Later, he told me, "I was really trying to give it to the other half [his partner], but he was in no mood. A few more 'ums' and 'ahs' on my part, and I would have been home free!" (Had he hesitated a bit more, Bryna implied, he would not have had to perform this difficult procedure.)

This was not the only time I observed patients distrustful about the youth of their potential surgeons. Perhaps we should be working on a reverse Grecian Formula, I joked, where instead of turning gray hair back to its original color, our formula would give young surgeons gray hair, making them look older and more experienced. No, Bryna said, he used to feel terrible when patients thought he was too young, but no longer. Somehow, all the patients who switch from him to his senior partner because of his youth seem to be the cases where they have trouble; these are the patients who have complications when Hamilton operates on them. It's just chance, he said, but it has happened so many times now that he no longer feels bad when they prefer Hamilton.

As we waited, Bryna told me that his car, a BMW, had just been rear-ended and totaled. "I really loved that car!" he said regretfully. Another sporty car, I thought, remembering that Bryna's partner drove a Porsche. I noticed that Bryna smoked cigarette after cigarette when he was not with patients; his partner had told me that he used to smoke, but had given it up. I wondered if Bryna wore seat belts; his partner refused to use them, as did many of the other surgeons I had talked with. (I asked Bryna about the seat belts later; he had started using them three weeks before the recent accident, because a new law mandating their use had just been passed.)

As we began to make patient rounds, Bryna telephoned the operating room to find out what time the operation was scheduled for. The head operating-room nurse first promised him a room at 1:00 P.M.; the time was postponed until 2:00, then 2:30. As we went from room to room, visiting his hospitalized patients, Bryna kept calling the operating room, emphasizing the emergency nature of the case and pressing the head nurse to provide a room as soon as possible.

We visited six patients, including Dr. Thomas, the retired dentist who had been operated on that morning, and a woman in her twenties who had come into the emergency room with a stab wound made, said Bryna, by a "poltergeist." "She says she doesn't know how it happened," he explained with comic relish. "She doesn't know who did it." She was "all coked up" when she arrived at the emergency room; they used to get a lot of cases like that in the inner-city public hospital where he was trained, he said.

After finishing rounds, we sat in the doctors' lounge, chatting with the other doctors who entered and left and making periodic calls to make sure an operating room would be ready as soon as possible.

At 3:30, Mrs. Gordon was on the operating-room table. After anesthesia was administered, Bryna "prepped" her, himself—residents usually do this task—shaving her pubic area, painting her abdomen with an antiseptic solution, and draping her body with blue operating-room sheets so that, eventually, all one could see was the abdomen. Bryna was assisted by a resident, whom he instructed with great patience, although the young man appeared clumsy and unskilled. Later, the chief resident "scrubbed in"; he moved quickly and competently and the procedure began to flow more smoothly. Two nurses and an intern also assisted.

Bryna and the first house officer carefully opened the abdomen in layers until they reached the large bowel, which was enormously distended. Bryna made a small incision, placed a suction tube in it, and attempted to empty out the feces that filled the intestine. Usually, the patient has several days to prepare for such an operation, and the bowel has been emptied beforehand through diet and enemas; but this is impossible in an emergency. When the patient is obstructed, as was Mrs. Gordon, more stool than usual is present, since the patient has been unable to evacuate naturally for some time. Performing an emergency operation on a colon filled with stool is not only messy and unaesthetic; it is dangerous, since the stool can contaminate anything it touches with bacteria that may subsequently cause infection.

It took almost two hours for Bryna, assisted by house officers and nurses, to empty the large intestine. The tube kept clogging; it had to be repeatedly unclogged, spilling feces, or exchanged for another tube. The circulating nurse kept running from the room to get more tubes. Everything that touched feces or touched something that touched feces—such as the tube—was contaminated, or "dirty." The scrub nurse could not touch anything contaminated without contaminating her sterile gloves (which then would have contaminated anything she handed to the surgeons). "Dirty" blades, sponges, and tubes had to be disposed of separately, apart from other waste products. It was a long, messy, smelly task. Despite occasional expressions of impatience or distaste when feces spilled, the surgeon, house officers, and nurses were remarkably patient and worked steadily until the bowel was finally emptied.

The surgeons scrubbed again and continued. Bryna felt inside the incision with his hand, off to the patient's right, and said, "Damn! Damn! Oh, damn it to hell!" "Liver mets [metastatic lesions on the liver]?" inquired the chief resident. "Yeah," said Bryna, who then brightened, saying, "Maybe it's a cyst!" After exploring further, he said, "It's involving the small bowel, too."

Bryna had arranged to have his office hours, scheduled for midafternoon, begin at a later hour. As the operation continued, the office hours were postponed to a later and later hour. Finally, at 5:10, when it was apparent that the operation would go on for some time, Bryna asked a nurse to telephone his office and cancel the hours. His partner, Hamilton, sent a joking message from the operating-room lounge, volunteering to finish the operation so Bryna could hold office hours. "He hates office hours," explained Bryna, returning a message inviting Hamilton to go to the office and see Bryna's patients for him.

Bryna and the chief resident removed a section of small bowel with a lesion in it. They joined the two edges of remaining bowel by hand, a procedure I had observed infrequently; most of the surgeons at Rice Community Hospital used a stapling device to perform this "end-to-end anastomosis."

After joining the edges of the small bowel, Bryna felt in the abdominal cavity and reported that the gallbladder was filled with stones. "Stones and badness," said the chief resident, who also felt the gallbladder before they removed it. It was enormous and very black. The liver was "studded" (Bryna's phrase) with multiple cysts, or lesions; they removed one for the pathologists to study. "Path" (as the pathology department was known) was already closed; the pathologists kept nine-to-five hours and would have to examine the lesion the following day. The two surgeons used an electric cautery to stem the bleeding from the liver, which bleeds copiously when cut.

The surgeons then removed a large section of large intestine. "Let's identify where we're coming from and where we're going," Bryna said, working slowly and painstakingly. He checked every nook, cranny, and crevice within the abdomen with his gloved hand. The operation, which had been scheduled as an "exploratory laparotomy for obstruction," was eventually listed on the patient's chart, as a "sigmoid colon resection, small bowel resection, cholecystectomy, liver biopsy, and colostomy."

Bryna finished the major portion of the operation at 8:00 P.M. leaving the chief resident to attend to the final details. Because the large amount of feces present during the operation increased the possibility of infection, the surgeons left the top layer of the abdomen open; this facilitated monitoring and controlling for infection.

Most surgeons I observed went to talk with the patient's family while the house officers finished the final "closing," which requires less skill than the rest of an operation. Bryna waited. He explained that he had once told a family that a patient was all right while the house officers were attending to the final details, and three minutes later, the patient had "coded" and died. Now he talks to families only after patients have reached the recovery room and their condition has stabilized. Instead of leaving the house officers to complete the final details, Bryna waited in the hallway, looking into the operating room occasionally. He quietly watched the patient being removed from the table before leaving.

While we were waiting for the house officers to finish, I asked how Bryna had known Mrs. Gordon had lost weight, when she had not mentioned the fact. She just looked as though she had, he replied; she probably had other symptoms as well, which she had ignored because she wanted to visit her son in Hawaii. How did he know it was cancer? Bryna went to the refrigerator outside the operating room, took out the plastic bag containing the section of sigmoid colon they had just removed, which was waiting to be inspected by the pathologists the following day, and indicated a hard spot, explaining that this was a cancer lesion. He cut into it, showing what it looked like, and then pointed out the "apple-core" lesion that had blocked the bowel.

We entered the recovery room adjoining the operating-room suite, glanced at Mrs. Gordon, who was beginning to wake up, and then went to talk with her husband, who was in the hallway outside the operating room. It was approximately 8:20 P.M. Dr. Gordon had been waiting since 2:00 P.M., when his wife had been brought to the operating-room suite on a stretcher to await a free room. Bryna led the husband to the patient lounge, gently asked him to sit down, sat next to him, and clearly and compassionately explained just what they had found: obstruction, apple-core lesion, lesions in the small and large bowels, possible spread to the liver. He spoke with directness and clarity, treating the veterinarian as a colleague. When Gordon questioned him, Bryna drew a diagram to explain matters more thoroughly. The husband was very quiet and seemed to grow smaller as Bryna talked. "What do you tell the patient?" Gordon inquired. "I tell her I found and removed lesions, but that I won't know for sure what it is until the pathology report comes back, which is technically true," said Bryna, "although I'm pretty sure it's malignant." He explained that Mrs. Gordon would look very different when her husband saw her: after major surgery, she would be very pale and sick-looking, with tubes coming out of her. I did not recall hearing another surgeon explain this change in appearance to family members.

After leaving the husband, Bryna said in a pitying tone, "He's destroyed!"

He then returned to the recovery room to check the patient's condition and call her internist to discuss the results of the operation. Then, back he went to the husband to talk with him some more—he wanted to see his wife before going home—and then back to the recovery room, where Bryna coaxed the nurse in charge into letting Dr. Gordon come in for a minute to see his wife. "Let's clean this act up!" said Bryna briskly to the nurses, helping them straighten Mrs. Gordon's bed and arrange her hair and gown before her husband saw her.

Later, he explained that he is able to get things done at Saint Augustus in ways that are impossible for him to achieve at Rice Community Hospital. He has been at Saint Augustus for years, and his senior partner was there even longer; everyone has known him since he was a house officer, when he worked there for some time. He said that the busiest and most influential surgical group at Rice can probably bend the regulations a bit there, as he can at Saint Augustus.

During the operation on Mrs. Gordon, a nurse had taken a phone call for Bryna. There was a possible "AP" [appendicitis] in the "ER" [emergency room], and the patient's medical doctor—in this case, a general practitioner—wanted Bryna's opinion. Bryna had told the practitioner to ask his senior partner to make the consultation when a second phone call informed him that Dr. Hamilton was too busy to see the patient. He instructed the nurse to say he was in the middle of an operation and that they should find another surgeon. But, when we left the recovery room with Dr. Gordon, who had squeezed his wife's hand and said a few words to her, we learned that the possible case of appendicitis was still waiting in the emergency room. It was 9:15. Bryna had not stopped for lunch (he never does, he said) nor had he yet eaten dinner. We went down to the emergency room, where the patient, an eight-year-old boy, had been waiting for three hours. The parents had heavy accents. "You're Polish!" he said. They said they were. "My mother is Polish," he told them. After feeling the child's abdomen and stating that it could not possibly be appendicitis, Bryna telephoned the boy's general practitioner. He noted that the child had a fever and abnormal white count, said he might be suffering from a virus, and recommended that a pediatric resident see the boy. He promised to arrange for this. Bryna telephoned to ask for a pediatric resident, waited until she arrived, and then introduced the resident to the family before leaving the emergency room.

We again visited Dr. Thomas, the dentist he had operated on that morning. It had been a very simple operation, said Bryna, but there had been a few complications, probably from the patient's heart medication, and he wanted to make sure everything was all right. Dr. Thomas complained that he was unable to sleep because of the noise of the ventilator attached to the patient in the next bed. We walked to the nurse's station, and there Bryna coaxed the nurse into agreeing to move Thomas to a new room. He then told Thomas he was changing rooms.

Back we went to the recovery room for a last look at Mrs. Gordon. Holding her hand, Bryna talked with her. She asked what they had found. "Lesions," he responded, telling her where the lesions were located. He said they would not know exactly what the lesions were until they received the pathology report in about four or five days.

At 10:15, Bryna changed and went home for dinner.

THE BURDEN

Dr. Bryna is the surgeon many people seek: well trained, technically skilled, confident, and compassionate. In the best of all

possible worlds, his virtues would have no cost; they would
be considered, as indeed they are in a certain sense, priceless.
Yet, certain costs are exacted, from Bryna and from his
family.

Time

Let us examine Dr. Bryna's day in more detail. Bryna arranged
to meet me at 8:00 A.M. at Rice Community Hospital, where
he probably intended to make rounds on his patients before
the operation at Saint Augustus, which was originally scheduled for 9:30. Did he begin rounds there at 7:00 A.M.? I did
not think to ask, but many surgeons do. The Saint Augustus
operation was moved ahead to 8:30, which means that his
partner, Dr. Hamilton probably made—or completed—rounds
for him at Rice. This coverage is one advantage of a partnership; if Bryna had been in solo practice, he would have had to
visit his patients at Rice after finishing at Saint Augustus.

Whenever he started, this much of his day's schedule is
certain:

8:30 A.M. operating-room suite, second floor
Operation on Dr. Thomas.
10:45 A.M. recovery room, second floor
Dictate notes, check on Dr. Thomas, receive telephone calls,
chat. The recovery room adjoins the operating-room suite,
so Bryna could go through the OR suite to reach the recovery room without entering the outside hallway. (This
means he did not have to cover his "greens" with a white
coat to guard their sterility or put on a freshly laundered
and sterilized scrub suit after leaving the operating-room
suite.)
11:20 A.M. emergency room, first floor
Examine Mrs. Gordon. The emergency room is some distance from the operating-room suite, in another building,
connected by winding corridors.

11:40 A.M. emergency-room waiting room, first floor
Talk with Dr. Gordon. The waiting room is across the hallway from the emergency room.

12:00 P.M. emergency room, first floor
Phone calls for barium enema and to find a surgeon for second opinion.

12:20 P.M. radiology department, first floor
Barium enema for Mrs. Gordon. Radiology is quite some distance from the emergency room.

1:00 P.M. emergency-room waiting room, first floor
Tell Dr. Gordon his wife needs operation.

2:00 P.M. surgical wards, second and third floors
Make rounds on six patients, including Dr. Thomas. The patients' rooms were some distance from one another, on two floors.

3:00 P.M. doctors' lounge, first floor
Chat with colleagues, smoke, drink coffee (available in an urn), phone operating room several times.

3:15 P.M. operating-room suite, second floor
Change to sterile "greens" in doctors' dressing room, scrub hands in sink outside operating room.

3:30 P.M. operating room
Operation on Mrs. Gordon.

8:00 P.M. operating-room suite, hallway outside operating room
Observe house officers finish operation.

8:15 P.M. recovery room, second floor
Check on Mrs. Gordon's condition.

8:20 P.M. hallway outside operating-room suite, second floor
Bring husband into patient lounge off hallway, tell him about operation. The patient lounge is next to the operating-room suite but some steps from the recovery room.

8:35 P.M. recovery room
Check Mrs. Gordon's condition (second time), telephone her internist.

8:45 P.M. patient lounge
More words with Dr. Gordon.

8:50 P.M. recovery room, second floor
Talk nurse into allowing Dr. Gordon in to see wife, help nurse arrange wife's bed, hair, and gown before husband enters (third time Bryna sees her after operation).

9:15 P.M. emergency room, first floor
See boy with possible appendicitis, telephone general practitioner, arrange for pediatric resident to see child, introduce resident to family.

9:45 P.M. Dr. Thomas's room, surgical ward, second floor
See Dr. Thomas (for third time after operation).

9:55 P.M. nurses' station, surgical ward, second floor
Talk nurse into changing Dr. Thomas's room.

10:05 P.M. Dr. Thomas's room, surgical ward, second floor
Tell Thomas he is moving to new room.

10:10 P.M. recovery room, second floor
See Mrs. Gordon (fourth time), briefly discuss findings.

10:15 P.M. operating-room suite, doctors' dressing room, second floor
Change from "greens" into business suit. Home for dinner.

On this particular day, which if not "average," was certainly representative, Bryna worked from 8:30 A.M. to 10:15 P.M.—almost fourteen hours, perhaps longer. Like many successful surgeons, he may keep such hours five days a week, and on occasion, six or even seven (Bryna and his partner take turns being "on call" on weekends—for emergencies and rounds on their hospitalized patients). This is a heavy burden of work.

Space

My second point—which is so obvious to doctors they don't even notice it, and is invisible to patients and families, who see their surgeons at one point in time and space—is just how much physical ground Bryna covered during the day. Like

Saint Augustus, many hospitals are composed of several buildings of various ages, connected by long, mazelike corridors that are usually traversed at a half-run by hurried surgeons and house officers. Their first year at a new hospital, house officers learn the quickest routes from one spot to another, including the most convenient stairways. Surgeons rarely bother with hospital elevators, which are invariably slow; stairs are frequently taken two at a time. Most frequently, Bryna covers this much ground at two hospitals, Rice Community and Saint Augustus. Some days he operates at both hospitals; he may have to drive back and forth between the hospitals several times to operate, make patient rounds, and on occasion, examine patients (like Mrs. Gordon and the child with possible appendicitis) whose internists or general practitioners want a surgical consultation. In addition, Bryna and his partner occasionally see patients and operate at a third hospital in the area when specifically asked to do so by the patient's "medical doctor" (the term used for doctors who are not surgeons). This extends the driving and walking to a third location, since daily rounds must be made on such patients until they are discharged from the hospital. Bryna and his colleagues stride back and forth, through winding hospital corridors, up and down hospital stairs, from operating room to radiology to emergency room to patients' rooms. They cover a lot of ground, fast, but many slow down when they reach patients' rooms. (One surgeon described how, when he was being trained by the celebrated cardiac surgeon, Dr. Cooley, and made rounds with him on as many as fifty patients, Cooley would run from room to room, then stroll into the room "as though he had all the time in the world.") Bryna's work, then, requires an enormous expenditure of physical energy, not only when operating, but in the daily details of patient care.

The Emotional Burden

Bryna expends psychic energy as well. Let us examine his behavior during the day. As the chief resident said, Dr. Bryna is a compassionate surgeon, who displays exceptional empathy and respect for patients. He is also remarkably conscientious.

First the compassion. Bryna introduced to me the retired dentist he had operated on in the morning as "*Doctor* Thomas"; he also acknowledged the profession of Mrs. Gordon's husband, treating the retired veterinarian as a colleague and addressing him as "Doctor." Many surgeons disregard the status and titles of other health professionals. Bryna's care for the titles reflected his care and regard for the *persons,* in painful and difficult situations, where illness, fear, and impersonal hospital routines tend to strip patients and their families of status and identity.

When he spoke of losing three patients, including a seventy-two-year-old man, as "tragedies," and again, when he noted that a patient's husband was "destroyed" after learning she had cancer, Bryna risked a kind of closeness to the emotions of families that few surgeons allow themselves. In surgery, tragedy becomes routinized: every day, every patient, every risk, involves an actual or potential tragedy. I found that when, after several weeks away, I returned to the hospital, I was struck anew by the profound tragedies that fill surgeon's lives; even as an observer, my feelings became blunted, perhaps in self-protection. Somehow, Bryna's feelings do not seem to have become blunted.

I once observed Bryna visit two patients dying of cancer. Outside the first room, he remarked, "It's hard to find things to say every day, it's so tragic!" But he entered, chatted with the patient, and said reassuringly, "I'm here every day. I see you every day." When the second patient pleaded, "Stay with me," he replied, in a soft, warm tone that carried complete conviction, "I told you I'll stay with you, and I'll stay with you!" Many doctors find it frustrating and painful to see patients they cannot help. As hope vanishes, doctors may gradually, almost inconspicuously, drop dying patients from their hospital rounds. Such interaction is particularly difficult for surgeons, who seek rapid and positive results. As one man declared, "I'm a surgeon. I do surgery. I don't view it as my role to be a caretaker!" When I questioned surgeons about who handles their postoperative care, Bryna responded: "Patients fall into two categories. In the first, the end result of the postoperative care is healing. . . . I follow the patient a few weeks, and then they're discharged to their medical doctor. The other class is cancer patients. They stay with me till they die." His response was unique.

When he delays talking to families until patients have reached the recovery room and their condition has stabilized, Bryna exhibits a mixture of compassion and conscientiousness. Most surgeons allow senior house officers to "close" the patient and finish the final details on their own—this seems to have become their unofficial prerogative—and take advantage of this time to talk to family members. Bryna was considerate of the house officers: he observed them inconspicuously from a hallway and did not breathe down their necks, as though he distrusted their abilities. He was, however, close enough so that he could step in if an emergency erupted. Bryna also demonstrated compassion and conscientiousness when he explained to Dr. Gordon what his wife would look like after a serious operation; managed to get him into the recovery room to say a few words to her; and helped the nurse to clean her up to improve her appearance for the husband's visit.

At 9:15, after working for more than twelve hours, Bryna went down to the emergency room to see the child who had been waiting for three hours. He could easily have asked a surgical house officer to see the boy—residents are available around the clock—and request that he be summoned from home to operate if the house officer thought the child had appendicitis. Bryna had not eaten all day and was hungry—he devoured the better part of a box of cookies provided by the emergency-room nurse. However, he examined the boy himself; established common ground with the undoubtedly frightened parents by mentioning that his mother was also Polish; took the trouble of telephoning to arrange for a pediatric resident to see the child (rather than requesting that the nurse or surgical resident call the pediatric resident); and waited until the resident arrived so that he could personally introduce her to the family. This shows kindness as well as conscientiousness.

One may argue that seeing the child demonstrated good business sense. General practitioners and internists feed patients to surgeons; taking good care of those patients keeps the supply coming. Thus, when Bryna called Mrs. Gordon's internist after the barium enema and again after the operation, he was not *only* being considerate. His attentions, however, went far beyond the bounds of business sense.

The Mental Burden

Bryna is unusually painstaking. (His senior partner told me he had offered Bryna a job when he was a house officer because he was so extraordinarily conscientious.) Taking pains involves not only an expenditure of time and energy, but also a kind of disciplined alertness, an intense concentration on each case and what can be done in advance to avoid difficulties. After operating on Dr. Thomas and Mrs. Gordon, he saw each four times that day. He telephoned the operating room before Mrs. Gordon's barium enema to warn that he might have an emergency procedure that day and kept telephoning, every half hour or so, to keep the pressure on, so that the head nurse would give him an operating room as soon as possible. He arranged for the barium enema, asking for the most competent radiology residents by name, observed the procedure in person, and quietly arranged for a senior radiologist to assist when the residents appeared to be having difficulties.

He prepped Mrs. Gordon for the operation himself, rather than leaving this task to the nurses and house officers, as do many surgeons. (This is one way for a surgeon to assure that everything will be done right, but not every surgeon takes the time and trouble to do so.) He was painstaking during the operation; his emphasis was upon carefulness, not spectacle or speed, checking every nook and cranny within the incision a number of times, to ascertain how many organs were involved in the spread of cancer and to be sure they had removed as much diseased tissue as possible. He joined the ends of the small bowel by hand; some surgeons contend that this "hand-done anastomosis" is superior to using a stapler (and it also demonstrates Bryna's technical facility).

Discussing caring and conscientiousness, a house officer said of Bryna: "He takes endless pains. He seems to think you just can't take too many pains."

My account may make Dr. Bryna sound implausibly perfect, even saintly. Not so. For one thing, he is a *young* surgeon; he had been in practice four years when I observed him, and still had much to learn. His partner noted that Bryna does not know how to manage his time as well as an older, more experienced doctor; he chatted on the telephone and in the doctors' lounge during the day I spent with him, rather than fitting in other tasks to shorten his work day. When Miss Washington began to complain and wriggle during her operation, a more experienced surgeon might have known how to quiet her or induce the anesthesiologist to do so. Rather than exhibiting the icy and effective composure of his senior partner, Bryna became tense and lost his cool. He has a cruel sense of humor and is intolerant of surgeons he believes to be incompetent or pretentious; he was responsible for some ferocious practical jokes, crushing remarks, and unpleasant gossip about people he does not respect.

Bryna is, however, an extraordinarily caring, compassionate, and conscientious surgeon. When I inquired about Mrs. Gordon six weeks after her operation, Bryna's partner showed me a clipping from the local newspaper. After leaving the hospital, she had sent the newspaper a letter, nominating Bryna as their "Man of the Year." She wrote: "He possesses all those qualities you wish for in your doctor—concern, compassion, confidence and just a general T.L.C. [tender loving care] manner. He commands the respect of the nursing staff and his colleagues, as well as of the patient."

The Costs for His Family

Bryna went home for dinner at 10:15 P.M. What of his wife, holding dinner until 10:30? What of their child, who is usually sleeping when he arrives home? Bryna said that his wife, a former OR nurse, understood his work and sympathized with what he was doing. I should like to hear her version. What does she tell the child about why Daddy is not present to enjoy triumphs, help discipline infractions, and contribute to the texture of family life? How does she feel about their social life as a couple, curtailed because he arrives home too late or too tired to socialize and is frequently forced to cancel engagements at the last minute? Bryna belongs to the most successful group at his hospital; it is possible that he earns "megabucks," or will do so in the future. He has little time to spend them, however. Do they console Mrs. Bryna for the loss of her husband's company? Does the respect of the community—which she undoubtedly enjoys—compensate for having to hire people to help with small household tasks (installing storm windows, moving furniture, repairing appliances)? Is she disconcerted when friends, acquaintances, and repairpeople giving estimates, make snide comments about "rich doctors"? Perhaps she would prefer Bryna to the megabucks; Bryna might choose his wife's company to the megabucks, as well. Neither is given the choice. If he is successful and dedicated, he pays the price. So does his family.

Critics might point out that Bryna has chosen this life; he might choose to see fewer patients, to be less busy. This apparently simple decision is difficult to implement, however. Successful doctors in private practice who wish to limit their patient load do so with difficulty. They cannot turn down colleague referrals without the possibility of turning off those referrals entirely. It is not easy to say no to a previous patient, a patient's family member, or even a patient's desperate friend, who seeks a caring, compassionate, competent surgeon. Naturally, Bryna and his partner might find a third surgeon, to lighten their patient load. This has its own problems, however. The two men must have complete confidence in the new partner; they must be convinced that the new surgeon has sufficient surgical skills to give their patients top-notch care and sufficient interpersonal skills to keep those patients happy. As many dedicated doctors have told me, choosing a partner is as difficult, perhaps more difficult, than choosing a spouse. One spends more time with the partner, and one relinquishes something very close to one's heart to that person— one's patients. If the partner has less technical skill, less judgment, less character or compassion, one's patients will suffer; if that partner is less "patient-prone," one's practice will suffer. Many doctors, perceiving these potential difficulties, prefer long hours to the gamble of a new partner.[1]

The Malpractice Threat

Bryna may accept the costs, most of the time. He is doing work he loves; he is successful in his profession; he is admired by patients and respected by the community. He makes a more than comfortable living (as one doctor said to me, it's nice "to do well from doing good"). Mrs. Bryna, who knew much about a surgeon's life before they married, may also share his dedication.

On some occasions, however, Bryna does resent the time, effort, and care he devotes to patients—when he cares for strangers who have come to the emergency room and is sued for his pains. Bryna described a malpractice suit he was involved in. A young woman was brought into the emergency room after an automobile accident when he was on call. She was quadriplegic when she arrived, and nothing could be done to reverse it. The family sued—for twelve million dollars—charging the surgeon and hospital with responsibility for her quadriplegia. "It's very impressive to get a letter from your malpractice [insurance] company, telling [you] that you're covered for one million dollars," said Bryna, [and informing you that] "you have to protect your assets and get a lawyer, because they may take them." Some doctors, less conscientious than he, avoid their turn on "trauma service." Bryna, too, was threatening to refuse to cover the emergency room. The case had not yet come to trial, and Bryna knew the jury might ignore all issues of negligence and law and decide to compensate the young woman for her ruined life and hopes. No matter how they are decided, such suits exact a high price.

6

LET'S GO FOR IT!

By push of bayonets, no firing till you see the whites of
their eyes.

Frederick the Great

In medicine, sins of commission are mortal, sins of omission venial.

Theodore Tronchin

*S*OMEONE HAD blocked out the "FE" on the "FEMALE LOCK-
ERS," where women (doctors, nurses, and female anthropologists) change to sterile green scrub suits to enter the
operating-room suite. That morning, I went back and forth
three times between two doors, both bearing the legend,
"MALE LOCKERS," before the joke became evident. At Mountain
View Hospital, as in all hospitals I observed, you enter the
lockers from the public hallway. Unlike many hospitals, however, the Mountain View lockers exit directly into the OR
lounge. After changing into "greens," you must walk through
the lounge to reach the actual rooms where operations are
performed. The OR lounge, containing armchairs, a table, a refrigerator (where nurses store lunches and snacks), and a coffee machine on a counter (frequently bearing cookies, cakes,
pizza, and other caloric offerings), is a fine place for an anthro-

pologist to sit and check out the surgical action. Senior surgeons, house officers, anesthesiologists, and nurses congregate here, smoking, chatting, telephoning, eating, drinking coffee, and waiting for operations whose rooms or personnel are not yet free.

At 11:00 A.M., Dr. Sylva and the chief resident, Raoul, were seated in the lounge, waiting for an operating room in which to perform a partial colon resection on Mr. Joseph Rocco, age seventy-five. The photocopied operating-room schedule for that day—containing the name of the surgeon, the house officers who would act as first and second assistants, the patient's name and age, what operation was planned, and the time the procedure was scheduled for—listed the operation for 10:30. But, the one room containing the straight stirrups Sylva preferred (to hold the patient's legs as they operated) was occupied, so the surgeons were waiting for the surgeon using it to finish, and for the aides to clean and sterilize the premises.

I waited with them. A colon resection is a fascinating operation to observe. It's a pleasure to view the complex inner architecture of the abdomen—so exact, so beautiful, so finely designed, it might well persuade an atheist of the existence of a prime shaper and mover. Watching surgeons' skills being challenged is absorbing. A surgeon must have patience and dexterity, to manipulate and explore all those yards of bowel; knowledge and technical mastery, to locate and remove the affected portion of bowel; clinical acumen, to decide (after observing the bowel and receiving the pathologist's report on the portion that has been removed) just what procedure to perform on the remaining bowel; knowledge and skill, to staple or sew the edges to each other (or to extrude one edge through the abdomen, giving the patient a temporary or permanent colostomy); patience, knowledge, and clinical judgment to ascertain that everything that should be removed has been removed. The operation is sufficiently complex so that, although general surgeons have traditionally performed it, a new specialty, that of colon surgery, is beginning to emerge. At Mountain View Hospital, it was the chief resident, with more than four years of surgical training, who had the privilege of acting as first assistant at colon resections, and on occasion, performing all or part of the procedure under the supervision of the attending surgeon. Sylva, too, enjoyed colon resections; he had the reputation of "stealing" them from his junior partner, Dr. Kim (of performing as many as he could, leaving the less interesting and skilled procedures to Kim).

"Where are all the medical students?" inquired Sylva. "Why do they spend all their time being lectured to by the chief, when they could be seeing the real world?" Sylva contended that book learning and journal articles were a poor substitute for hands-on surgical experience, and that his thirty-five years of such experience made him a better teacher than the chief, who, although he operated on patients, had never engaged in the private practice of surgery. The two surgeons discussed giving the patient a temporary colostomy (where a portion of the severed colon is put through the abdominal wall, so that the patient's stool empties into a bag) and Sylva told Raoul that his aged Italian patients, like Mr. Rocco, tolerated colostomies poorly, finding them dirty and humiliating.

Sylva, who usually complained about being kept waiting, was in a good mood. He recounted two smutty jokes, observing his female audience, composed of young nurses and the anthropologist, to see if he had succeeded in eliciting a blush; sang the air force anthem enthusiastically and off key, and talked of his service in the marines during "the real war, the big one."

The operation began at 11:30. When the scrub nurse handed him the wrong instrument, Sylva said in a loud, angry voice: "Damn it, I said small mets [Metzenbaum scissors], not large! Can't you do anything right!" The young woman turned pale; her eyes glistened, but she did not cry. A few minutes later, Sylva asked her, in a soft voice, "Did you get sick when

I yelled?" I think it was his form of apology, although he "yelled" a few more times during the operation.

Sylva and Raoul worked rapidly. Both were known for their technical facility. Few words were needed; Sylva would begin a gesture and Raoul would finish it. The harmony, grace, and efficiency of their movements were a pleasure to observe. As they cut, Sylva sang tunelessly, "Off we go, into the wild blue yonder . . ." When they cut into the colon, Sylva paused, looked at it appraisingly, and said, "I gotta evaluate this and see if I've got the guacamoles to put it together."

After the two surgeons removed a large portion of bowel and sent it to pathology for analysis (pathology said it was an abscess), Sylva said in a half-teasing tone, "You don't know what's in my mind!" Raoul replied, "I know what's in your mind, and I'll go for it!" With speed and dexterity, Raoul and Sylva then joined the remaining edges of bowel to each other, using a special device to staple the edges together. Sylva and I then left the room, as Raoul and the intern closed the patient.

It was 1:00 P.M., and there was another procedure I wanted to observe. The patient was already on the table, but the attending surgeon said there was time for me to get a snack before they began to operate. As I consumed coffee and a roll in the cafeteria, Sylva joined me at my table. "Where's the chief?" he inquired. "I don't know," I replied. "I'm not studying the chief, I'm studying senior surgeons like you." "Oh, you want to learn about *real* doctors!" he responded. People like the chief [full-time academic surgeons, who have never been in private practice] don't really know how to do things, he explained. "None of them could do what we did today. They would have done three separate procedures on that poor old man, subjecting him to three anesthesias." First, they would have given him a colostomy, Sylva said; then, in a separate procedure, they would have "taken down" the bowel [operated on the bowel and removed the abscess]; finally, in a third procedure, they would have repaired the colostomy. Dr. Kim, his partner, would probably have done it in two procedures: the colostomy and bowel, and later, the colostomy repair. He said of his partner and colleagues, "Oh, he'll criticize me, they'll all criticize me!" He indicated that only he has the nerve and skill to dare to do something like this; that's because he has thirty-five years of experience and he's fast. "Raoul is fast too, isn't he?" I asked. "Too fast, sometimes," Sylva responded. "Did you notice how I took over sometimes and did things myself, or suggested how he should do things? He's very good, though," he said. Could he have done it this way with Craig? I asked, mentioning another senior house officer (whose colleagues joked about his lack of technical facility). "No, Craig isn't quite ready for operations like this," said Sylva. I told him that one of the house officers had said that he, Sylva, had "golden hands." His partner, Kim, has good hands and is fast, said Sylva; of course, he trained him. (Kim had been a house officer at Mountain View Hospital, where Dr. Sylva had been an attending surgeon for thirty years). "You can train people, but aren't the hands a given?" I inquired. Well, he spots good hands, responded Sylva. He can tell how new house officers are going to do the minute they come into the hospital.

Sylva's partner, Dr. Kim, joined us at the table and asked about the operation. Sylva described the abscess they had removed. Kim formed the extended fingers of each hand into a circle, moving his hands apart, then together a few times, so that the circle made by the edges of the fingers of one hand touched the circle made by the edges of the fingers of the other. He was inquiring, wordlessly, whether they had joined the two edges of bowel together (performing a "primary," or "end-to-end," anastomosis, rather than the colostomy that originally had been discussed). "Yes, that's what they did!" I said. Sylva explained, "It was clean and we worked very fast, so we didn't have to do a colostomy." His partner responded by very slowly crossing himself twice.

Four days after the operation, while making morning

rounds at 6:30 A.M. in the intensive care unit with the surgical house officers, I saw Mr. Rocco, looking lively and well oriented. To Raoul's apparent astonishment, the patient was taking liquid nourishment rather than being fed intravenously. Sylva had come in, seen how well the patient looked, and ordered it for him. The chief joined us in the intensive care unit, and Raoul and he discussed Mr. Rocco's case. "Well, it has a 70 percent chance of success." said the chief in an ironic and self-distancing tone. "Yes," replied Raoul, "but he has renal failure and diabetes; it might be more than a 30 percent chance of failure." Raoul sounded as though he disapproved intensely of what had occurred. (This was surprising. During the operation, I had recorded Raoul's words: "I know what's in your mind, and I'll go for it!") "The worst thing," said the chief, ruefully, "is that if it works, it will encourage Sylva to do more things like it!"

Two days later, Mr. Rocco was transferred from the intensive care unit to "the floor." The following day, a week after the operation, he was back in the intensive care unit, pale, unresponsive, and very sick-looking. The house officer who presented the case to his peers during morning ICU rounds described it as "Dr. Sylva's aggressive resection with a primary anastomosis." Mr. Rocco was a "septic patient" (meaning infection was present). The big question, discussed by the residents, was: did his anastomosis (the joining of the bowel) leak?

Later, in the cafeteria, I heard Sylva say with great vehemence to his partner, Kim, "There's no leak in that anastomosis! I'm *sure!*" With some difficulty, Kim managed to persuade him they should perform a diagnostic procedure to indicate whether or not there was a leak.

After a week's absence from the hospital, I noticed during morning rounds that Mr. Rocco was no longer in the intensive care unit. When I asked a junior house officer what happened to him, he responded: "He died last week. He had fulminating *Clostridia*." He added, "That operation should never have been done on him." (The house officer explained that "*Clostridia*" are bacteria that can infect the bowel and that "fulminating" means sudden, severe, and with a rapid course.) Later that day, I heard Raoul say that Mr. Rocco's case would be presented at next week's M and M conference.

Every Friday morning, Mountain View Hospital holds a weekly surgical mortality and morbidity conference, where statistically unexpected or clinically interesting deaths and complications are discussed. Attendance is mandatory, and surgeons and house officers sign a sheet of paper passed around the room. Although every surgeon does not attend every conference, someone who misses too many is sanctioned. Surgeons make a special effort to attend conferences where their cases are discussed. Theoretically, an M and M conference is the forum for the free and frank discussion of difficulties and errors among peers.

The following Friday, however, the surgical house officers who presented cases for discussion did not mention Mr. Rocco. Instead, the surgeons considered two small, relatively unimportant cases in exhaustive detail. The discussion was elliptical; I understood little of what was going on. After the conference, I asked a senior house officer, who had recently begun talking quite openly and frankly with me, if he would explain just what had been occurring. Why did Mr. Rocco go unmentioned, when his case involved significant issues? Why, instead, were two relatively unimportant cases discussed for a full hour? My friend and informant (or, as he liked to put it, my "mole"), Yehuda, verified what I was beginning to suspect. The important thing in M and M conferences at Mountain View Hospital, said Yehuda bitterly, was not what was said but what was *not* said. Thus, the significant cases, Mr. Rocco's and another, where serious issues were raised, were postponed. And in the two cases that were discussed, people hinted but never said that the first case concerned a technical error: a clip was improperly placed. As for the second case, said Yehuda, the patient never should have been operated on. The referring endocrinologist was in error; the surgeon should never have removed the organ, at least not all of it; they performed the wrong operation and injured the nerve, as well. None of this is mentioned at the M and M's, said Yehuda. People hint that a mistake was made, but no one points a finger and says it straight out. He confirmed that this was why I found so many of these conferences confusing and a bit boring. No one says the endocrinologist was mistaken, he said. If someone did, the endocrinologist might not refer more cases to that surgeon. No one says a surgical colleague was mistaken. People just hint. At a university hospital, reported Yehuda (who had trained for two years at an elite university hospital in another country), they would criticize what was done wrong and jump on the person who did it. At Mountain View Hospital, it's all a whitewash, he said harshly.

The following week, Mr. Rocco's case was presented at the M and M conference by a second-year resident. As a radiologist placed Mr. Rocco's films on a light box, the house officer began in classic fashion: "This seventy-five-year-old white man was admitted on November 15. Early in his admission, he was diagnosed as suffering from diabetes mellitus. He had left abdominal pain. It got worse, and a surgical consult and a GI [gastrointestinal] consult were called. GI films were taken on the twenty-first, a barium enema given on the twenty-second." "It was probably a diverticulitis abscess," said the radiologist. Sylva kept arguing with the radiologist, insisting he was not showing all the films; the radiologist disagreed, saying he had taken the films and knew what was there. "Sylva thinks they're presenting this case just to embarrass him," whispered Yehuda, who was sitting in front of me.

The resident continued:

Dr. Sylva operated on the twenty-eighth. The abscess was seen, a left colon resection was performed, well out of the field of the abscess, and an end-to-end anastomosis was done. The patient was given intravenous alimentation one day after the operation, and on December third, was placed on a full liquid diet. The night of the fourth, he had foul-smelling urine; his BUN and creatine rose. A urine analysis was positive for lots of white cells and bacteria. A gastrographic study was obtained as an emergency measure seven days postop. There was no evidence of a leak at the anastomosis [the joining].

"The films showed a walled-off collection," said the radiologist, pointing. "It was a giant divertic [diverticulitis]," said Sylva. A technical discussion ensued. Raoul, the chief resident who had assisted Sylva, said nothing.

The house officer presenting the case reported that the patient had fulminant *Clostridia* and that he "coded" for the second time on December sixth, and died. He cited some literature on *Clostridia* and noted again that the patient suffered from renal failure and diabetes. The question was, he said, did the patient have interabdominal sepsis [was infection present in the abdomen]?

Sylva said: "A primary resection was done because we judged step by step that we could get away with it. And we *did* get away with it!"

The discussion continued. A young attending surgeon, Dr. Raina, known for his mild manner and encyclopedic knowledge, kept questioning Sylva. Sylva lashed out at him, disagreed with him, tried to ignore his questions. Quietly and stubbornly, Raina continued questioning. The chief, who frequently disagreed with Sylva at M and M conferences, used irony to make his points about the unwisdom of Sylva's actions. Sylva ignored the chief and his opinions. Everyone talked at once. Sylva's angry and excited voice rose above the others, making it difficult to hear what was going on.

A quiet voice emerged from the back of the room. The room silenced. Dr. Johnston was one of the most respected and admired surgeons in the hospital. Although he did most of his operating at another hospital, where he had been an attending surgeon for twenty-five years, Johnston was well known at Mountain View Hospital. Doctors and nurses frequently asked him to operate on their families—a high compliment. Johnston was perhaps the only surgeon I never heard Sylva disparage—or contradict. This was the first time I heard Johnston utter a critical word during an M and M; he usually held himself somewhat aloof from hospital politics and disagreements.

Said Johnston, with quiet authority: "I question the operation you did in the face of an abscess. You should have drained the abscess and done a colostomy." He added, "Waiting five days to operate was inexcusable!"

Although Sylva did not confront Johnston, he kept defending himself, insisting there had been no leak in the joining [anastomosis]. "If there had been a leak, I'd have had my head between my legs!" he declared.

One of the questions raised was the source of the clostridia bacteria. Did the bacteria come from the gastrointestinal tract? The patient had had bacteria in his urine before surgery. Did his abscess contain *Clostridia*? An internist who specialized in infection stood up and gave a brief lecture on *Clostridia*. He said the patient should have been operated on as soon as he entered the hospital; they should not have waited to operate.

Almost every attending surgeon at Mountain View Hospital was present—a rare occurrence for M and M conferences. And, for the first time in my experience, the discussion extended beyond 9:00 A.M. Usually, when M and Ms threatened to run overtime, surgeons would start trickling from the room. No one left. Everyone had something to say.

Even when the conference was officially terminated by the chief, surgeons and house officers stood in the hallway discussing the case. I had asked my friend Yehuda to explain the issues afterwards. With the young attending, Dr. Raina, who had questioned Sylva so persistently, we adjourned to a small lounge frequented by surgical house officers and attendings.

When I told Raina that, in his quiet way, he had said exactly the same thing as Dr. Johnston, Raina responded, "Yes, but they listened to *him*!" Raina said that Mr. Rocco should have been operated on earlier, and that it was the wrong operation; the chance of complications goes from 5 percent to 40 percent when one operates on a left bowel without doing a colostomy. The patient started getting sick when he was still in his hospital room, before being returned to the intensive care unit, said Raina. His surgeons could have "gone back in" [reoperated to see what was going on] then, he said. When the patient got sicker, it was harder to reoperate and explore what was wrong. Raina and Yehuda pointed out that the infection might have come from the abscess, which could have been drained beforehand by his surgeons. When I mentioned Johnston's outburst, Yehuda remarked, "Yes, he gets fed up about once a year and says something!"

More house officers joined us. They were discussing surgical cases and techniques when Sylva entered the lounge and began to talk about Mr. Rocco. He insisted that the patient had not gotten *Clostridia* from the anastomosis [joining] and that the primary resection they performed [joining the edges of the bowel to each other, instead of giving the patient a colostomy] had nothing to do with his death. "Well," said Raina quietly, "he should have been operated on earlier." "I agree!" responded Sylva. "We wanted to. But the medical man [internist] refused. We really tried, and discussed it with him, but he refused and put a note on the chart. If we had operated and he died, it would have been *our* fault in case of a malpractice suit. This way, it's the medical doctor's fault. None of you have been in practice," he said, looking at Yehuda and Raina (who had just gone into practice in July and had seen very few patients). "You've *got* to do what the referring physician wants if he insists. That's the way it works if you want any more patients from him."

As Sylva started to leave the room, he repeated that he thought they should have operated immediately. Raina assented, remarking: "Yes. The sun should not set on undrained pus!" Sylva poked his head back into the room, inquiring, "Want to watch a master do a really fabulous operation?" "Yes!" I said. But Sylva was not addressing me. He was talking to Raina and Yehuda, who excused themselves and remained in the lounge.

Sylva's operation was complex, involving three separate joinings (anastomoses) of the intestine. Sylva performed most of it himself, letting Craig, the resident whose technical ability was disparaged by his peers, do only bits and pieces, and watching and correcting him very carefully. At one point, he felt the intestine and said: "Oh, it's tumor, it's tumor! What a shame! He's going to go down the tube fast." He spoke with real feeling. Sylva's partner, Kim, entered the room and asked if he could help. Sylva responded that he did not need help. Later, he inquired: "What is it? Am I getting senile or something, that everyone wants to help me?" The young scrub nurse was new. When she handed Craig a special stapler that had been used once, she asked if it needed to be refilled. No one heard her. When Sylva noticed that the stapler had not been refilled, he scolded the nurse for carelessness in a loud, angry voice. "I asked you if it should be refilled," she rejoined loudly, and Sylva exploded. "Don't you yell at me, young woman," he bellowed. "I don't allow that! Perhaps these young men will, but you've got to know your place!" No one moved, no one said a word, as Sylva continued, loudly criticizing her lack of respect, sense, and propriety. Soon afterwards, another, more experienced nurse entered the room and quietly relieved the young woman Sylva had screamed at. I did not notice if she was crying. Sylva told the new nurse, in a belligerent tone, that she could file an incident report if she wanted, but that nurses had to know how to behave properly. When the operation was nearly finished, however, and the two house officers were closing the patient, Sylva went off to, as he phrased it, "kiss" the young nurse he had screamed at.

Later that afternoon I was talking to the chief in the OR lounge when Sylva entered and sat next to us. In an adjacent operating room, Raoul was prepping a patient for an operation Sylva was scheduled to perform. "Do I have to go in the room when Raoul opens?" he inquired. "Do I have to be there at all during the operation?" "No," responded the chief, "not so long as you're here [to be called in case of difficulties]. What is it?" inquired the chief. "A colon resection," responded Sylva.

When told about Sylva letting Raoul do the kind of case he usually "steals" from his partner, my husband said: "Well, he was just told that he killed a patient. That's no small thing. You know how terrible I feel, and how long I feel terrible, when I make one small mistake that might endanger a patient. You can't blame him for not wanting to do the same operation that killed Mr. Rocco, right after the M and M."

Before we examine the implications of Dr. Sylva's behavior, let me emphasize that I have altered a number of significant details to avoid identification of the surgeon, the hospital, and the patient. I have done my best to retain the medical, social, and emotional valence of what occurred but, inevitably, much is lost in translation. As a result, surgeons who read this account may feel that the case does not "ring true." They will be correct. The case is only partially true. I must, therefore, caution doctors: you cannot read about Mr. Rocco's symptoms and his treatment as though this were a technical case awaiting your diagnosis. Because so many details had to be omitted or changed, the medical history and its social implications are truncated. The case, as recorded in my field notes, is richer and more understandable than the story presented here. But, legal and moral constraints shorten and oversimplify my story.

Now, let us consider Dr. Sylva. Sylva is a Prima Donna, the most recognizable character in the surgeon's morality play.

Volatile and high-strung, he was an expert at keeping people off balance. Once he screamed at me so loudly during an operation, I had difficulty remaining calm and not weeping (I had injudiciously relayed a telephoned message from his office, while he was operating); he apologized, indirectly, an hour or two later. Another time, when I was wearing what I thought was a particularly elegant dress, he grinned at me and said, "Your bra's showing!" It was not, but he managed to make me lose my composure.

Sylva's flamboyant self-confidence bordered on grandiosity. When asked if he had ever known anyone during his career who typified his ideal surgeon, Sylva's response was simple: "My ideal surgeon? *Me!*" He was a handsome man, who dressed well. He flirted with women and attempted to dominate men. He could be charming, annoying, impossible. But he could not be disregarded. He was a very high-profile person; everyone knew when he was on the scene.

Sylva had impressive technical facility. He was daring to the point of recklessness. He loved to operate. And he was convinced that his daring, skill, and experience allowed him to break the rules that more prudent and less skilled surgeons were bound by.

Sylva plays another role at Mountain View Hospital. "He's one of the last of the Old-Time Surgeons," said his partner, Kim. "There's only one other left in the mountains." "The last Old-Time Surgeon left in North America!" is how the chief of surgery characterized Sylva, with combined relish and rue. Complex diagnostic tests and technology were unknown in the old days; instead, surgeons relied on experience, intuition, daring—and personal knowledge of each patient. A surgeon's son in practice with his father, whom he described as "an old-time physician-surgeon," noted that both Sylva and his father "look at the patients, not just the numbers [test results]." He said that when he was a house officer at Mountain View Hospital, they used to hate to make rounds with Sylva. "He didn't teach, he visited with his patients. They were all his friends; he'd ask them about their families and everything." Old-time general surgeons did every operation in the book; their competition was the general practitioner, who also performed surgery, not the surgical subspecialist. Specialized teams were rare; the Old-Time Surgeon was flying by the seat of his pants, winging it across uncharted territory.

The autocracy of the Old-Time Surgeon extended beyond the operating room. A surgeon, described somewhat wistfully how, during the Depression, his surgeon-father would announce to a patient: " 'Roberta, you've got cancer and you're going to lose your breast. And you'll have to pay for your operation in advance.' And that's just the way it happened!"

Sylva and Kim had the busiest surgical practice at Mountain View Hospital. When Sylva had an emergency and wanted to "add on" an unscheduled procedure, the operation occurred within a few hours—even when another surgeon's procedure had to be "bumped" to give him a room. His cases were scheduled for the morning hours and most frequently occurred on time: he rarely had to wait for an operating room. The chief also was accorded these informal prerogatives, but many surgeons were not. Some were kept waiting while a more influential surgeon's case was substituted for their own. Some had difficulty scheduling procedures—even semiemergencies, which should have been performed the same day. In the hospitals I studied, this informal control over the OR reflected the power and influence of a surgeon.

Sylva's power and influence may explain why Raoul, the chief resident, seemed to be playing a double game, encouraging Sylva's behavior at the operating table, then deploring it to the chief. Raoul would be going into private practice the following year. He planned to stay in the mountains, and Sylva's enmity could damage his career. (Sylva was a dangerous enemy; I had seen him virtually ruin the career of one young surgeon who had offended him, and seriously injure that of another, who had clashed with him.) On the other hand, if Sylva liked Raoul, he might send him a few small cases. If Raoul did well with these, the satisfied patients would send their friends—and thus, a surgical practice grows. Raoul was even more dependent on the chief's goodwill than on Sylva's. The chief could recommend him to a prestigious program for subspecialty training, if Raoul felt he needed this to give him a competitive advantage in the area. The chief could also, if he wished, find a part-time job for Raoul for the first year or two after completing his residency, to help him meet his office expenses and the high costs of malpractice insurance, before his practice started to pay for itself. Raoul's motivation is unknowable, but his behavior was clear: he agreed with both men, and affronted neither.

Sylva had grown up in the mountains; his father had been a general practitioner (and he had a daughter in medical school, who planned to become a surgeon). The parents of many of his patients had been cared for by his father. He attended medical school with the most successful internist at Mountain View Hospital; they had been friends for almost forty years. The internist "fed" patients to Sylva. "He's the goose that laid the golden egg," said Yehuda. He told me that Sylva often did not even look at his patients' X rays. "He acts almost like a workman, not a doctor," said Yehuda disapprovingly. "He does just what the internist tells him needs doing." Sylva's younger partner was trained at Mountain View Hospital; the younger internists, who were house officers with Kim, fed *him* cases. My impression was that the Sylva group cared primarily for working-class patients; Dr. Johnston's and the chief's patients, on the other hand, appeared to range from working-class to upper-middle-class. Sylva knew his patients intimately; he'd inquire with real warmth and interest about their parents, children, aunts, and uncles. When interviewed, he described how he convinced an unwilling patient to have an operation he believed was necessary:

You should sit down; don't stand up. Sit at their level, talk at their level. Don't talk like a professor; show a lot of concern. That's not difficult—surgeons have concern for the patient. Your appearance is important. You shouldn't be all disheveled, your hair should be combed, you should dress well. Twenty years ago, if I didn't gain their confidence it was because I was too young. You lay it down in their language and give them the confidence that you're the best thing that ever happened to them. It's like making love to a woman. *Seriously*! The most important thing is a feeling of true concern.

But Sylva made errors. On occasion, grievous errors. As in this case. A surgeon who reviewed this case for me said that Mr. Rocco probably had diverticulitis, an infection of a small sac in the wall of the colon (large bowel). The infection was either localized in an abscess (a collection of pus) in the peritoneum or spread throughout the peritoneum. The operation on Mr. Rocco's left colon was dangerous because the patient had diabetes, which made him particularly prone to infection, and because the left colon tends to have more bacteria and more dangerous bacteria than the right colon (because stool remains in the left colon for several days before being eliminated through the anus). When infection is present, an operation on the left colon is that much more dangerous. One way the dangers are minimized is by giving the patient a temporary colostomy: a portion of the severed colon is put through the abdominal wall so that stool empties into an external bag, rather than joining the two remaining edges of colon together within the abdomen. A colostomy is considered safer in an infected environment.

Sylva contended that his anastomosis (the joining of the edges of the bowel) did not leak and spread infection into the abdomen. This is quite possible: Sylva was a consummate technician. But even if the anastomosis did not leak, infection may have already been present in the bowel. Such infection can cause the suture line (the stitches or staples that join the edges of the bowel to each other) to "break down"; the joined ends of the bowel get infected and begin to open, further spreading bacteria from the abscess and the colon.

The *Clostridia* bacteria, causing the infection that killed Mr. Rocco, quite possibly came from the abscess. If the surgeons had drained the abscess ahead of time, the subsequent colon operation might have been less dangerous. A left colon resection would still have been more dangerous than a right, especially on a diabetic patient, but at least the operation would not have been performed with known infection present.

Sylva claimed, when talking with Raina and Yehuda, that he had wanted to drain the abscess but that the patient's internist opposed this and wrote a note to that effect on the patient's chart. This, he said, made *him* liable for a malpractice suit if he had gone ahead and drained the abscess and something had gone wrong. The general surgeon I consulted agreed: "That's really serious. If there's a note on the chart, and something goes wrong, *your* neck is out in the guillotine." This surgeon noted, however, that deciding not to drain the abscess in such a case would be a *legal* decision, to avoid a possible malpractice suit, and a *financial* decision, to encourage further referrals from the internist. Medically and ethically, said my consultant, Sylva was obliged to do whatever he believed was best for the patient, no matter what the opinion of the referring internist was and no matter what the internist wrote on the chart. A second surgeon I consulted expressed skepticism. "It doesn't sound right," he said, indicating that an internist might well ask the surgeon to drain the abscess and do nothing else until the patient's condition had improved sufficiently for his colon to be operated on. The consequences of an undrained abscess are so serious, said the second surgeon, that he just could not understand why the internist insisted on *not* draining it. "It doesn't make sense!" he exclaimed. (Raina's remark that "the sun should not set on undrained pus" is a well-known surgical adage. In this case, GI (gastrointestinal) films were taken on November twenty-first, a barium enema was performed on the twenty-second—at which time Mr. Rocco's doctors would have known he had an abscess— but the abscess remained undrained and the patient was not operated on until the twenty-eighth.) The story may *not* have made sense; Sylva may have been rationalizing his behavior after the fact. He had a reputation at Mountain View Hospital for rationalization and blaming everyone but himself when something went wrong. Whether or not Sylva was telling the truth about the internist and the note on the chart, not draining the abscess was a serious *medical* error, and if it was done to pacify the internist or avoid responsibility for a potential malpractice suit, it was a *moral* error as well.

Few people in the hospital would discuss Sylva's errors with me, and those who did would say a few words and then change the subject. I was therefore unable to learn just how long he had been making such errors and whether they had increased with age (he was in his late sixties). I suspect they had. It was Dr. Johnston who had told me that the hardest thing for a surgeon to know is when he should stop operating. "You don't lose your technical facility." he said. "You just lose—well, your attention span gets less, you can't concentrate in the same way for the same amount of time." I wondered whether he was referring to Sylva but did not ask.

The chief of surgery at Mountain View Hospital was aware of Sylva's errors. "He has a high rate of complications," said the chief. He advised Sylva, he argued with him, but he never took him on in a head-on collision. The chief had been at Mountain View Hospital for ten years; he had been recruited from the Midwest, and Sylva had been on the search committee that offered him the position. Unlike Sylva, the chief, an intelligent, erudite, kindly man, did not relish controversy. If he had challenged Sylva directly, he might well have lost. Sylva knew the members of the board of trustees. His father had practiced at Mountain View Hospital before him, and his

wife was related to a powerful local politician. Sylva was embedded in the area, in the local and hospital power structures.
It would be a brave, perhaps reckless, man who would take
him on.

The surgical house officers knew of Sylva's errors; they
were a subject of gossip on the hospital "grapevine." Kim occasionally let something drop that made me think he was quite
aware of what was going on. But no one had the power, authority, or perhaps courage to take him on and attempt to force
him to retire. Sylva talked of retiring. Several times a year, he
and his wife would take long trips, leaving the practice to his
partner. But he always returned—and resumed "stealing" the
most interesting operations from Kim.

Retirement for surgeons involves more than merely leaving
one's work. One leaves one's identity, one's "self" as well.
Surgeons spend many years being trained; when they go into
private practice, they work long hours, with little time off.
With the exception, perhaps, of golf, few practicing general
surgeons I met had hobbies or outside interests. Their physical, social, and psychic energy goes into surgery, which offers
them physical, social, and psychic rewards. They are identified, by others and themselves, primarily as surgeons. I heard
an anecdote once about a famous surgeon: Watching an older
man operate badly, the celebrated surgeon said to his assistant,
"When I get to that stage, promise to tell me." Many years
later, the assistant did tell him that he was losing his touch and
should consider retiring. "Shut up!" responded the surgeon.
The story may have been apocryphal, but the sentiment is recognizable. Surgeons have invested too much in becoming and
being surgeons to contemplate giving it up with equanimity.
("I feel like an amputee!" confided a surgeon who had recently
retired.) Many surgeons find it difficult to cut back, to operate
less frequently, or to confine themselves to less interesting, less
challenging procedures. And, as patience and judgment falter,
a surgeon's arrogance may fill the void.

Did Sylva perform the primary anastomosis on Mr. Rocco, reconnecting the bowel rather than giving the patient a colostomy, because he lacked patience and concentration? Probably not, because surgeons tell me that, in these circumstances, it is easier to give the patient a colostomy than a primary anastomosis. Nevertheless, his behavior may reflect a more subtle kind of impatience: he performed the spectacular, risky procedure, rather than stopping to reflect about what might happen if he failed. He did not *think;* he acted. I believe Sylva suffered from hubris, from the overwhelming belief in his own magical powers to confront fate and defy the law of averages. Once, when Raoul "jokingly" called him a gambler, Sylva responded: "No, you guys are gamblers. *I'm* a lucky surgeon!"

Dr. Raina and Raoul discussed the odds of Sylva's "getting away" with joining the ends of Mr. Rocco's bowel together, rather than giving him a colostomy. Such odds are known; surgical journals publish studies where various procedures are measured against one another, with the resulting complications and survival rates expressed statistically. The chief stressed this literature and insisted that his house officers be familiar with the latest studies, procedures, and statistics. Sylva denigrated the chief's "literary" bent; he claimed that his thirty-five years of operating on thousands of patients had taught him more than he could learn from journal articles written by academic surgeons who spend more time experimenting and writing articles than operating. (Sylva's skepticism about the statistics presented in academic studies, and his overweening confidence in his ability to beat the odds, may not have been entirely unjustified. The studies published in journals aggregate the results obtained by many different surgeons; the studies contrast *procedures,* not surgeons. A number of surgeons told me that a technically gifted surgeon can indeed change the odds in his favor. The question is, how far can he change the odds?)

Sylva chose to "go for broke," to stake everything on one spin of the roulette wheel—to try for a probability, however small, of succeeding with one procedure, rather than taking the prudent route of performing three separate procedures, which he contemptuously said the chief would have done. Yes, the patient would have been subjected to three separate anesthesias, which had their own statistical probability of complications. And yes, it would have been less interesting, less challenging, less daring to go that route. But in this case, the law of averages prevailed. The gamble failed. Sylva's "luck" ran out and the patient died.

Why did Sylva behave as he did? One difficulty with anthropological research, as opposed to writing novels (where one can compose motives as one invents behavior) is that in the observed world, motives are essentially unknowable. A researcher who is working on a classic "hate doctors" book has a simpler task than mine. That researcher can take it for granted, without reflection, that Sylva was animated by the worst possible motives: venality, stupidity, and a kind of blind, stiff-necked pride. He may have been. But, even if he were, the situation is not as simple as many medical critics would have it. Social scientists, who often criticize laypersons for ignoring the social context of behavior, frequently forget this context when they discuss doctors. As an Old-Time Surgeon, Sylva did not perform in a social vacuum: he cared primarily for old-time patients. Old-time patients differ as much from modern patients as do old-time from modern surgeons. One day, I made rounds with a young surgeon, who was somewhat embarrassed when an aged Italian man kissed his hand. This patient's view of his relationship to his surgeon was similar to Dr. Sylva's view: *both he and Sylva took it for granted that the surgeon knew what was best for the patient.*[1] Such a patient does not resent a God-like surgeon; he would not have another.

A social scientist colleague who heard this story expressed distress, saying:

> I can understand that some patients hate colostomies. And perhaps Sylva's working-class Italian patients really would have pre-

ferred to have him join the edges of the bowel, whatever the risk. After all, a seventy-five-year-old man may have preferred risking death to having to empty his feces from a bag several times a day. But why didn't the surgeon ask? Why didn't he sit down with the family and discuss the whole thing, tell them the odds—he surely could have expressed it in terms they would have understood—and asked what they wanted him to do?

If I were a patient, I would want my surgeon to discuss these issues with me. So would my sociologist colleague. Indeed, so would every medical critic and bioethicist who deplores the arrogance and paternalism of doctors, surgeons in particular.

What I do not, and cannot, know is whether Mr. Rocco and his family would have preferred such a discussion. What would a seventy-five-year-old, working-class Italian man, who felt a colostomy to be dirty and humiliating, have decided? Would he have wanted to be put in a position where he was forced to declare, "I'd rather you let me die than leave me attached to a bag filled with my ———?" Would his family want the responsibility of such a decision, of having to say, "We can't cope with Papa like that, it's better you let him die than do something like that to him."

Sylva, as I said, was embedded in the community. He is not the only doctor in the area whose father cared for the families he cared for, whose daughter or son may eventually care for their children. Sylva belongs to the same moral and social community as his patients. They attend the same church. If he had given Mr. Rocco a colostomy and the patient had been miserable, the whole community would have known of it. Rocco would have called Sylva and complained. The patient's wife and children might have called. They would talk about Sylva and the terrible thing he did to their husband and father. Here we have the relationship between the old-fashioned doctor and his patients that many are so nostalgic about. The doctor knew his patients intimately. The patients knew their doctor. They belonged to the same face-to-face community.

This embeddedness in the same social matrix imposes constraints as well as opportunities.

Medical critics frequently call for regulations and panels of inquiry to supervise what they perceive as the endemic misbehavior of doctors. But, it must be noted that such generalized regulations are applied to *particular relationships* between doctors and patients. An old-time doctor who has intimate knowledge of his patient may disobey generalized rules and then be sanctioned by outside panels who, ignoring doctor, patient, and social context, conclude that the doctor's behavior was medically incorrect—even when the doctor behaved as the patient wished, even requested. Personalized relationships have costs as well as benefits. So do generalized rules.

In this case, Sylva made the decision for Mr. Rocco. He did not ask; he acted. He went for broke and failed. Sylva knew he failed. Despite his bravado, he knew that his decision at the operating table resulted in a death. The death of a friend, perhaps, as well as a patient.

I do not contend that Sylva made the right decision. What I want to point out is that his motives were not necessarily, or primarily, base. Sylva is an Old-Time Surgeon, a Prima Donna, who assumes without question that he knows what is best for his patients. He is an anachronism. When we say that he should have consulted with the patient and family before risking everything on one spin of the roulette wheel, we are judging him by today's standards. Today's patients are more knowledgeable and insistent on sharing crucial decisions. Today's doctors are slowly changing to meet their demands. Although we may acknowledge that Sylva's motives were not necessarily horrendous, we can deplore his behavior and note that surgeons can no longer behave as he did and be sure to get away with it. (I do not know if the case resulted in a lawsuit, but it has the potential to do so.)

The day of the M and M conference, where Sylva's behavior was publicly criticized, the chief said to me, "Sylva thinks it's like the old days when he could do just what he wanted and no one questioned." Sylva did, in fact, do what he wanted. He was questioned, however, and sharply criticized by his most respected colleague. Sylva is no longer king of the operating room. Nor is he monarch of Mountain View Hospital. His behavior is no longer condoned. The chief did not prohibit him from operating, as perhaps a more autocratic and contentious chief might have done. But his days of operating are numbered. He will decide to retire on his own. Or be pressured, subtly or not so subtly, to do so. And the next generation of surgical Prima Donnas, such as Raoul, already perform under more constraints than Sylva ever experienced. Social change in medicine may be glacially slow. But it does occur.

7

DEADLY SURGICAL SINS

Virtue, then, is a state of character concerned with
choice, lying in a mean . . . between two vices, that which
depends on excess and that which depends on defect.
With regard to feelings of fear and confidence courage is
the mean; of the people who exceed . . . the man who
exceeds in confidence is rash, and he who exceeds in fear
and falls short in confidence is a coward.

Aristotle
Nicomachean Ethics

From avarice, there spring treachery, fraud, deceit, per-
jury, restlessness, violence, and hardness of heart against
compassion.

Gregory the Great
Morals on the Book of Job

THIS CHAPTER examines misbehavior. The surgeon's
ability to perform "miracles," the power he wields over
those in need, and the temperament of the miracle worker
each has its shadow side: the capacity willfully to do harm
rather than good. The chapter explores deadly surgical "sins,"
which I have arranged in four categories: vices of excess;
generative sins; defects, or character flaws; and deficiencies.

The classification can help identify appropriate responses to various kinds of misbehavior.

Unlike those critics who, perceiving the world as a simple opposition between good and evil, believe that a causal chain links surgical error to misbehavior, and misbehavior to bad results—all of which can be encompassed by the term "malpractice"—I find such issues complex and ambiguous. Misbehavior assaults patients, with trust betrayed, hopes blasted, miracles pledged and not performed. Misbehavior and malpractice (the two are related but by no means identical—see Chapter 6) pose exquisitely sensitive questions for surgeons as well, involving their deepest vulnerabilities: psychic, social, legal, and financial.[1]

In the early 1980s in the United States, when I carried out my fieldwork, the subject of surgical misbehavior was particularly disquieting. No longer the "naive subjects" of the seventies (who made little effort to conceal their misdeeds from inquisitive researchers),[2] surgeons were angry and apprehensive about the hostile and litigious climate encompassing them. Referring to this environment, many used the phrase "in this day and age," with comments like, "In this day and age, you gotta move a patient whose condition isn't stable to give her a CAT scan to document her condition" and, "I think you need, in this day and age in the state of California, a pathologist's report." "This day and age" created difficulties for researchers observing surgeons. (In one hospital, where the hospital review board had to approve my research before I could gain access to surgeons, a senior surgeon intervened to defend the study to a suspicious review board. He subsequently reported saying: "You're worried about her finding out where the bodies are buried. Forget it, it's me you should worry about; I *really* know where the bodies are buried!" Well, I did learn where some—but by no means all—bodies were buried.)

My findings about misbehavior were restricted: what I was

allowed to observe was limited; what was explained to me, even more limited. My faulty medical understanding was compounded, not only by their reluctance to explain but also by my strategic decision to ask few questions when I suspected misbehavior[3] and by my determination to alter and disguise important surgical and social details when describing cases.[4]

The ethical scheme I present here, then, is provisional; the analysis, heterodox; the categories ad hoc and incommensurate. Moreover, because I perceive more ambiguity in what I was allowed to observe than do researchers such as Millman[5] and Katz,[6] my perspective makes for a more complex picture, which is more difficult to formulate and portray than a simple and pervasive image of misbehavior. As a result, my data are incomplete, my formulations imperfect. Nevertheless, I believe this analysis is worth attempting. I know of no similar effort. It is a beginning, to be improved upon by those with more inclusive data. (When members of the hospital review board, inclined to reject my project, asked the senior surgeon who defended it what the research would do for the hospital, he responded that it would do nothing for the hospital but might do something for medicine. People are worried about how to get doctors to regulate themselves after they stop being house officers, he said, and this study might help us learn something about this. I take his implied moral charge very seriously: to provide data and interpretations that might help surgeons regulate themselves.)

VICES OF EXCESS

The first category of misbehavior is related to surgical virtues.[7] "Vices of excess" involve an intensification of valued and valuable attributes of surgeons' temperament, character, and ethos. A surgeon must manifest courage, confidence, nerve, and a supreme belief in his own powers. These qualities, however, must be balanced and informed by the art, craft, and science of surgery. The surgeon cannot subscribe to his own mystique, relying upon miraculous powers in lieu of knowledge, judgment, skill, and an obsessive attention to detail.

Defying the Odds

Let us return to the case presented in Chapter 6, where an Old-Time Prima Donna decided to "go for it." Operating on Mr. Rocco's left colon without performing a colostomy, Dr. Sylva ignored known and inimical odds of complications—odds that were increased by the presence of an abscess in the patient's bowel. Sylva staked everything on one spin of the roulette wheel and lost. The patient died.

Had the surgeon explained the risks to the patient honestly and in comprehensible terms—working-class patients know as much about gambling as do surgeons and sociologists—and the *patient* had then decided to go for broke, we would not question the decision. Wagering the life of *others*, says philosopher Hans Jonas,[8] is not justified in order to gain a good, even a supreme good,[9] but only to avoid a supreme evil. "Seeking to save that without which all else is deemed worthless, at the peril of losing all in the attempt, may be morally justified and even commanded," he says. What this means in this case is that were certain death the alternative, then *and only then* would it be morally justified for the surgeon to decide to defy the odds and go for broke.[10]

In Aristotelian terms, Sylva behaved recklessly, or rashly. He was given to the vice of excess, to the sins of the overbearing rather than the underbearing, of those who do not too little, but too much. While courage is essential for a profession that dares to "dismember the image of God," excessive courage in a surgeon careens out of control into recklessness and can be deadly.[11]

Sylva, who referred to himself as "a lucky surgeon," comparing himself to the house officers whom he characterized as "gamblers," relied upon his luck to reverse the odds in his favor. Sylva's wager failed, and his actions were criticized by those whose opinions he most respected: his colleagues.

Defying the odds is on a different level of analysis from, for example, hubris, which I have also categorized as a surgical vice. The first concerns *observable behavior* and *known statistics*, the second, an inferred temperamental characteristic that motivates behavior. One might argue, with some justice, that Sylva's hubris inspired him to defy the odds. My classifications are contestable; they are designed to be illustrative, not exhaustive.

Hubris

To explore the surgical vice of hubris, let us consider a case. Cases are complex, motives murky, psychic and surgical details obscure to an outside observer. Yet, despite the ambiguity and loose ends of real-life cases—as opposed to the ordered oversimplifications of an "ethnography of indignation"—we can, I believe, learn much from a surgeon's attempt to cure someone who might be described as a "chronic patient":

> "There's someone in every surgical group who gets the real nuts," proclaimed Chris, to his fellow interns. "And, Villar's the one. That patient of his, Sandoz, the male nurse, is driving me up the wall. I didn't mind him all that much until Friday, when he kept calling me, all day and all night, wanting one drug after another. He pokes carrots and celery into his ileostomy to block [it], then yells for drugs. The man's crazy! He's a real Munchausen. Why else would anyone have thirty operations? And why is he being done at Foothills when he comes from the peninsula, not far from the university hospital? He probably used up all the local hospitals," declared Chris. "Besides," he added, "Why doesn't Villar write permanent drug orders for him, if that's what he wants, rather than letting six house officers do it, each one differently?"
>
> Earlier that day, the intern had tried complaining to Dr. Villar,

who had dismissed his accusation that Sandoz suffered from Munchausen's syndrome, contriving symptoms to bring to doctor after doctor, hospital after hospital. The surgeon admitted that the patient was "crazy," that his disorderly behavior and incessant demands for drugs had antagonized all the nurses and house staff, and revealed that a psychiatrist was visiting Sandoz and administering calming medications. Nevertheless, the patient had a serious surgical problem, insisted Villar, which was caused by a motorcycle accident, exacerbated by poor surgical care, and complicated by drug dependency, which had developed during his protracted treatment. "Chris," declared the senior surgeon, "you have to learn to take care of people, whether you like them or not, hate them or not, crazy or not. Your job here isn't to wean Sandoz off drugs or be moralistic, but to give him what he needs and help get him better so he can get out and take care of his problems."

I remembered hearing Villar and his junior partner discuss the complexities of the case: a male nurse, an ex-addict, thirty operations, a pending lawsuit against the trucker who had hit his motorcycle. The day before Sandoz's operation, I followed Villar into his room and heard the surgeon announce delicately: "We're going to look at you from the back way." "Oh, a proctoscope," said the patient.

Two days later, Villar told me they had operated on Sandoz and "cleaned everything up." I wondered whether Villar was being optimistic, but the patient was subsequently discharged.

Two weeks after the patient's discharge from the hospital, Chris announced to the house officers, assembled for breakfast after ICU rounds, that Sandoz was hospitalized again. The previous Saturday, said the intern, Sandoz had come into the cafeteria, where Chris was lunching with another house officer, and kept telling them, as they tried to eat lunch, how he was "spilling shit all over." The patient had then gone to the emergency room where, according to another house officer, the staff made three mistakes: first, they let Sandoz lie down on a stretcher (they never should have done that, he said, then some nurse feels sympathetic and you can't get rid of the person); second, a resident gave the patient Demerol; and, third, another resident gave him Demerol. That was it, said the house officer, he's back in now.

The young surgeons discussed the case. They talked about the difficulties they had discharging Sandoz from the hospital and how Chris had wagered that he would be back in as soon as possible. One resident contended that Sandoz had to be treated, whether or not he was impossible, whether or not he was crazy: the man was sick and needed care. Another disclosed that the psychiatrist who had been seeing Sandoz talked of admitting him to the local psychiatric hospital. One resident faulted Villar for operating on Sandoz in the first place. He contended that the patient was no better off than before, that in fact, he was worse, and that no one who had all those operations has a good chance to be cured by another operation—all that scar tissue will interfere.

Leaving the cafeteria, I met Villar's junior partner and mentioned Sandoz's return to the hospital. "Oh, he's crazy," said the surgeon; "there's nothing we can do with him. He does everything to make it worse so he can get drugs."

Two weeks later, Chris told me that he had heard a banging sound from Sandoz's room the previous morning. "Oh no!" he reported that he had said, but although the patient was no longer his responsibility, Chris had entered the room and found Sandoz hitting his head against the wall.

After several weeks' absence from Foothills Hospital, I inquired about Sandoz, and Villar told me that when the patient got better, he couldn't stand it and "decompensated." He said that Sandoz had been admitted to the local psychiatric hospital.

Three months later, a house officer who moonlighted at the psychiatric hospital reported that he had encountered Sandoz there. The patient was bleeding from his scar, which had been healed when he was discharged from Foothills. "He's a self-mutilator," said the resident, in condemning tones.

Sandoz was possibly an addict who also suffered from Munchausen's syndrome. There was some suggestion that the psychiatric hospitalization after leaving Foothills Hospital was not his first. The patient was clearly in pain, terrible, soul-searing pain. Saying "it was all in his head" is a facile and unhelpful oversimplification; the patient had serious psychic *and* surgical problems, a combination that is difficult, often impossible, to care for. Sandoz's psychiatric disorder(s) amplified and complicated his physical symptoms; his physical problems fed into his psychiatric difficulties.

Why then did Dr. Villar, a general surgeon who practiced at a community hospital, as opposed to a superspecialist practicing at a university hospital, presume that he could relieve a patient who had not been helped by thirty previous operations? [12]

We cannot be sure of the answer. Perhaps it was venality: although the Villar group was one of the busiest at his hospital, another case *is* another dollar in the bank. It surely involved defying the odds: after thirty failures, the odds of success were not overwhelming.

I believe, however, that his cardinal vice was hubris—the desire to show that *he,* John Villar, had the knowledge and skills to repair what more than twenty-five predecessors had failed to remedy. I suspect that Villar could not resist the challenge: to clean up the mess left by the others.

Hubris might be perceived as an excess of the indispensable surgical virtue of self-confidence (the opposite extreme being diffidence).[13] Too much belief in oneself and one's abilities plays into the patient's desperate quest for miracles; the surgeon offers the miracle the patient seeks and apparently believes he can perform it.

This is not the first time we have encountered Dr. Villar. He is the man who carried out what he himself described as "psychiatric surgery" on a woman who had undergone multiple procedures for suspicious symptoms (page 2). Twice, then, we have seen Villar abet patients in an unrealistic search for a miracle. He is surely unwise—many would say reckless—in his choice of patients.

When Chris, the intern, accused Villar of always ending up

with the crazy patients, he described how, when as a medical student he worked for two surgeons, one man would screen patients before agreeing to operate, telling them what to expect and what he expected from them, while the second would operate "on anyone." Like Villar, said Chris, the second surgeon always got the crazy patients. Chris did not employ the term "crazy" in a diagnostic, psychiatric context; what he was referring to was Mr. Sandoz's insatiable demands and inappropriate expectations. Such patients seek a drug, a treatment, a procedure that will rapidly and definitively terminate their agony. (Able to do nothing to ease their suffering, nurses and house officers, who have devoted their careers to relieving affliction, detest these patients; the demands escalate, the staff's frustration increases, and anger and punitive behavior proliferates.) "Crazy" patients hope for miracles, expect miracles, demand miracles. When the surgeon Chris worked for as a medical student screened his patients, he refused to operate on those with unrealistic expectations, thus weeding out the "crazies." It was Villar who told me that a surgeon can be judged, not only by his successes, but also by the patients he turns down. If we measure him against his own criterion, he fails.

Is Villar reckless or dishonest? A colleague, engaged in an ongoing feud with Villar (whose judgment must therefore be regarded with some suspicion), characterized him as "a little bit slippery-slimy." He functions in what Yehuda, a house officer, called "a gray area." (Despite the fact that Yehuda was often very critical, he did not judge Villar all that harshly.)

Villar is a complex, intelligent, even brilliant man. Although busy and successful—he was one of the men who made the "megabucks"—he may no longer have found his work exciting. The operations he performed, I felt, did not really challenge his superior intellectual and technical capacities. Perhaps Villar should have been an academic surgeon, at the vanguard of surgical practice, teaching, and research. Or a trauma surgeon, whose days are charged with excitement.[14] As it was, I suspect Villar created his own challenges.[15]

Magical Surgery

If Villar's vice in operating on Mr. Sandoz is classified as hubris, his operation on Mrs. Morelli (page 2), whose symptoms were probably entirely psychiatric in origin, can be categorized as magical surgery. Although Villar used the term "Munchausen's syndrome" to describe the patient, a psychiatrist might diagnose her ailment as hypochondriasis, "that disease in which there is no disease,"[16] or perhaps hysteria. The patient's internist, driven to distraction by incessant telephone calls, visits, and complaints, may indeed have "turfed" her to the surgeons. Instead of flatly refusing to operate, or "punting" her to a university hospital, where a world-famous surgeon might have possessed sufficient authority to convince the patient to discuss her symptoms with a psychiatrist, Villar encouraged her search for a magical solution to her problems. Whatever his justification, his behavior was a surgical sin, violating an injunction against operating on patients one cannot help.

Villar's vice is wishful thinking, one extreme of the virtue of hope, or positive thinking, the other extreme being negativism. A sanguine, positive, "can-do" attitude ("be ballsy, do it!") is a surgical virtue, except when carried too far. The surgeon *must* be positive, he must believe he can walk into the operating room and make that patient better—and he must convince the patient of his powers. But he must only believe he can do what he is able to do. What he is able to do may be difficult, on occasion, to determine; the line between grandiosity and self-confidence, between wishful thinking and positive thinking, must be respected.

GENERATIVE SINS

What makes generative, or "capital," sins particularly noxious is their procreativity: they lead inevitably to additional sins.[17] Impelled by an attachment to a lesser "good," the sinner defies the supreme "good"; this attachment and his defiance generate "daughter" sins.

Venality

The venal surgeon subordinates what should be the supreme medical good, the welfare of his patients, to a lesser good, money. I have described the vices of excess as an intensification of the temperamental characteristics of surgeons (as presented in Chapter 2). Venality, too, can be perceived as an intensification—or perversion—of the business of surgery (as discussed in Chapter 4). Its generativity makes venality particularly lethal among surgeons: it engenders other varieties of misbehavior.

Small wonder, then, that critics so focus upon venality, suggesting that all, or almost all, surgeons in private practice perform unnecessary procedures for profit. Although I suspect that critics overestimate its prevalence, their appraisal of its malignancy is accurate. Many critics, however, overlook the capacity of venality to generate not only sins of *commission*, doing that which should not be done, but also sins of *omission*, not doing that which should be done. Thus, venality may engender carelessness, when a surgeon so concentrates his attention on the operating room (where the procedures for which he is reimbursed are performed) that he neglects the preoperative and postoperative care that insures the safety and well-being of his patient. Venality may encourage a refusal to operate on patients who cannot afford a surgeon's fees ("They biopsy their wallet and if there's no money, they dump 'em on the public hospital," said one man, describing his former colleagues' treatment of emergency cases).[18] Venality generates sins of omission not only among private practitioners of surgery, but also in prepaid health plans, where it may encourage authorities to neglect expensive diagnostic tests, postpone or exclude necessary operations, and provide second-rate diagnostic and surgical equipment.[19]

Venality is a difficult sin for an outside observer to identify. What one notices is a multiplicity of sins committed by a particular surgeon: defying or ignoring odds; taking unconscionable risks; "stealing" patients from colleagues and precipitously operating on people whom colleagues were observing, hoping to avoid an operation; giving patients little time and care outside the operating room; performing a large number of unnecessary—or at best questionable—procedures. The observer also picks up hints and gossip. People rarely make direct accusations, but comments about how someone needs a lot of money—for the tuition of several children at medical school or for elaborately wining and dining a bevy of mistresses—can be suggestive, especially when that surgeon's patients have an extraordinarily high rate of complications. When I heard direct talk about venality, it always referred to surgeons who practiced at another hospital or who were in another surgical specialty. General surgeons, for example, might discuss an ophthalmologist who performed lens implants on aged women suffering from Alzheimer's disease, or a neurosurgeon who refused to perform a CAT scan in his office on a nurse unless he was paid in advance. It seemed likely that surgeons who knew this much about colleagues distanced by hospital or specialty knew at least as much about their general-surgeon colleagues. They knew—but they were not telling the prying anthropologist.

I observed two general surgeons whom I believed to be venal. Both were the subject of gossip and disapproval by colleagues; each had been categorized by me as a Sleazy Surgeon. The association between the sin of venality and the role of

Sleazy Surgeon is not accidental: venality generates sleazy be-havior. Every example of what I suspected to be venality in my field notes involved a number of other sins. To give a brief example of a particularly chilling combination of rashness, ignorance, defying odds, and venality:

> A young surgeon at a community hospital performed a vascular procedure on a patient who was suffering from high blood pres-sure and an ulcerated foot and was in borderline renal (kidney) failure. Surgeons at a prestigious university hospital had refused to operate on the man, contending that his condition was too poor and the risks too high. Four months after the procedure, the patient was still hospitalized. He was demented due to lack of blood to his brain; both legs had been amputated because of lack of circulation; his remaining kidney had failed and he was on renal dialysis. A house officer who hated to scrub on the numer-ous procedures the surgeon was still performing referred to the patient, with rueful and grisly accuracy, as "Dr. X's meal ticket."

Pride, or Hubris

One of the medieval "seven deadly sins," indeed the capital of the "capital" sins, pride can lead the doctor to defy the odds or believe in his own magical powers and can thus be classified as a generative sin. Pride is particularly seductive because it is so close to that virtue of self-confidence, upon which successful surgery depends. Therein, it differs from rank venality.

Because I am convinced that confidence to the point of arrogance is essential in surgery, I have analyzed it in an Aris-totelian framework. Conceptualizing hubris as a vice of excess leads, I believe, to more effective suggestions for curbing it than what is likely to be a fruitless effort to extirpate confi-dence—and even arrogance—entirely.

Surgical critics may disagree. Critics find surgeons' arro-gance and egotism particularly galling, relating hubris to a kind of grandiosity that engenders unnecessary procedures.

Their views have a certain justice. The difference between the critics' approach and mine is more one of emphasis than content. Where I differ is in my estimate of the value of surgeons' arrogance and egotism: I believe they are necessary, except in excess, while critics condemn these attributes out of hand.

It is surely more parsimonious to classify hubris as a generative sin that initiates other varieties of surgical misbehavior. The reader is free to dissent from my taxonomy.

DEFECTS, OR CHARACTER FLAWS

Impatience and Carelessness

I tried classifying impatience as a vice of excess, then as a deficiency, but it remained troubling.

In Chapter 1 (page 19) I mentioned the obsessive patience a good surgeon must display; we saw this painstakingness in action when we followed Dr. Bryna, the Compassionate Young Surgeon. A surgeon must take endless pains: at the operating table; on "the floor," when making rounds; at home, when a family member, nurse, or house officer telephones with troubling information about a patient. Impatience resulting in carelessness can be lethal. Impatience is, of course, a state of mind, which must be inferred; carelessness is more observable. Let us return to my field notes, to a description of a colon resection performed by Dr. Auerbach, a young attending surgeon, Amin, a chief resident, and Jeff, a third-year resident:

> *Field Notes.* Jeff did lots of it, Amin the rest, with Auerbach watching and doing some parts. I couldn't be sure, but it seemed to me that Auerbach was impatient and not really careful enough. They kept trying to fit a round knob they used for telling what size stapler to use for the colon anastomosis [joining]. The stapler is called an EEA, which stands for "end-to-end anastomosis." The patient, Victoria Vito, age seventy-six, had a *very* narrow colon

and the smallest gadget wouldn't fit, even when Amin tried and tried, with great sure-handedness and what looked like expertise. All that happened was that the "purse-string" stitches [holding the severed edge of the colon closed] broke, and the edge of the colon ripped. Auerbach insisted on trying the EEA, nevertheless. He took it off [to the side of the room] afterwards to look for the two "doughnuts" [small doughnut-shaped pieces of tissue that remain in the device] that show a proper anastomosis was done, when Amin said, "Don't bother to look." Auerbach didn't understand and kept on looking, till Amin informed him that there was a big rip in the colon. They had to do it [join the edges of the colon] by hand. Amin and Auerbach disagreed on the technique. Amin, I think, wanted to do it the classical way I had seen him do with the chief, where they do the stitches all around, holding onto the threads, and then tie them [the threads] one after the other. Auerbach wanted to do the bottom from the inside and the top from the outside because it was "faster." Jeff and Amin did it Auerbach's way (it was his patient).

Auerbach left, while the two of them were closing, but dropped in a few times to check up. Amin wanted him to do something, couldn't catch what it was, he speaks so softly, but Auerbach discounted it; he didn't have the time, he had a consult. . . . (I can't be sure of this, but it seemed to me that Auerbach was taking the quick, easy, sleazy way out for everything.)

At one stage, Auerbach said something to someone about how "the EEA [stapler] malfunctioned" and Jeff snorted. The next time, when someone inquired [colleagues dropped in during the operation to observe and comment], Auerbach told them the patient's colon was too small for the EEA. I got the feeling Jeff disapproved of the *way* Auerbach used the EEA, but maybe I'm reading things into it. It's quite possible the colon *was* too small; after all, those sizing things [the knobs that determined what size stapler should be used to close the colon] wouldn't go in.

My evidence of Auerbach's carelessness included his (1) insisting upon using the special stapler (the EEA), when the patient's colon proved to be too narrow for the sizing knob, (2) not noticing that the EEA had torn the colon, (3) insisting upon what he himself justified as the "faster" method of joining the edges of the colon by hand, (4) refusing to do whatever it was Amin requested at the end of the operation because he was in a hurry. When I tried the next day to tactfully elicit Jeff's opinions about Auerbach's behavior during the operation, he was close-mouthed. All he would say was, "It wasn't a symphony." (Indeed it was not. The three surgeons did not function as a harmonious ensemble, and the rhythm, grace, and sureness exhibited on occasion when operations were going well were absent.) In the end, my assumption of impatience and carelessness was determined not only by what I *saw*, but also by what I already *knew* about Dr. Auerbach.

Attempting an Aristotelian analysis of Auerbach's "vice," we might characterize nerve as the virtue, with impatience at one extreme and irresolution at the other. This is unsatisfactory, however. Perhaps *some* impatience and carelessness could be so classified, but surely not the behavior of Dr. Auerbach in this operation. Such impatience is unrelated to surgical virtues; instead, it is better conceptualized as a *moral defect*, related to a lack of self-discipline.

We might classify impatience and carelessness as a "deficiency of painstakingness" (see pages 19–20). Unlike ignorance and incompetence, however, one senses that an element of volition is involved—that the surgeon, if he so wished, could easily take more pains.

The two surgeons I observed who exhibited the gravest and most consistent lack of patience and painstakingness were both venal. Each hurried from patient to patient, procedure to procedure, spending too little time and attention on the sorts of efforts that are inconspicuous to the patients whose welfare they help insure.

Impatience and carelessness are fatal sins, representing lethal character flaws in doctors—surgeons in particular.

Untrustworthiness

This attribute can also be classified as a moral defect, or character flaw.[20] It is a deadly surgical sin, however, only when it leads to carelessness. When a surgeon is *personally* untrustworthy, not coming through emotionally for a patient, but *professionally* trustworthy, being competent and obsessively painstaking about the surgical details, one finds an unhappy patient, who has been given cold, but technically correct, care.

Lack of Caring

As previously noted (pages 25–26), the term "care" has a dual meaning in medicine: caring *for* the patient's body (taking pains and being careful) and caring *about* that patient as a person. Lack of caring about the patient as a person can also be categorized as a character flaw—a flaw that is, unfortunately, exhibited by a number of competent surgeons. Like personal as opposed to professional untrustworthiness, to which it is perhaps related, lack of caring, although deeply disturbing, is rarely fatal per se.

In an attempt to measure caring *behavior* among surgeons (as opposed to verbal responses to questions about caring), I observed examples of "ambulatory surgery," where patients were awake during the procedure. I noted whether the surgeon acted as though the patient were asleep, ignoring questions, fears, whimpers, or whether he comforted and reassured his patient. Surgeons displayed a wide range of caring and uncaring behavior. Here are two cases, observed in succession. The first was a breast biopsy, the second, a removal of a cyst from the patient's hand:

> *Field Notes.* I got to the room where they do the ambulatory surgery and Verdi was doing a biopsy. He and the patient were talking about restaurants. "Listen, we're struggling very hard to make you look good now," said Verdi. "If I had put the incision

here, I woulda been done a long time ago." "Will I know soon?" asked the patient about the biopsy. "Yeah," said Verdi, "it'll be nothing." They conversed and he showed her what he did and how. (He went in through the areola, so the scar would be just about invisible, which is what I've generally seen him do.) Verdi included her in the conversation between the nurse, house officer, and himself (in what seemed like a matter-of-course fashion). He told her about how there would be a lump afterwards from the stitches, and they conversed throughout the procedure. The patient looked [at the incision], when he was almost finished. "I got a suit home; maybe you could put a hem on it?" she inquired. "My father was a tailor," responded Verdi. He got a phone call and came back and reported, "OK, it's benign, she [the pathologist] says." Verdi coughed, and he and the patient discussed smoking. No, he doesn't smoke, but his father smoked; he probably smoked many packs just being near him. There was conversation, real conversation, as the procedure went on. He said to the house officer, "You don't have to be Jewish to eat Levy's Jewish rye bread [an advertising slogan], and you don't have to be a plastic surgeon to use a plastic surgeon's stitch. As my friend Dr. Kalman says, you get breast cases from the beauty parlor." He then explained to the resident and the patient that women compare their scars and people want to go to the surgeon who produced the most beautiful scar.

✳

The next patient was for Dr. Whiting; I introduced myself to him [in the hallway] and asked if I could watch, and he said yes. The patient was a teary young girl, who was telling the nurse she wished she could be put out. . . . Whiting entered, didn't talk to her. Then he saw big tears leaking out of the corners of her eyes. "Crying? Scared?" he asked. "Let me tell you what we're going to do. We're going to numb that area; then we'll do it. It's not a big procedure," he said. He left the room; the girl was still crying. The nurse sprayed her hand with Betadine [an antiseptic], and the hand trembled, like an uncontrollable shiver. Whiting was answering a page [paged on the hospital intercom, he left the room], said the nurse. Another house officer entered, and the two of them [two house officers] started the procedure [the house officer who started to assist the surgeon, and the second]. Whiting entered and watched them. The girl whimpered and Whiting asked, "Does it hurt?" "A little," said the girl, and he directed the house officers to give her more lidocaine [an anesthetic]. The house officers kept on going, the nurse held her hand and talked to her. She groaned, and one house officer said very quietly, "Sorry." (Don't know if she heard him; it was almost as though he was saying it to himself.) She started really crying, and after a few minutes, they gave her more anesthetic. The house officers kept on working. They removed the cyst, saying nothing to her; they were discussing another patient and then discussing what they were doing. Whiting returned as they were closing; Whiting went to the phone and talked [with his back to the patient and the room]. He then left the room. The house officers finished and with the aid of the nurse took the patient from the [operating] room toward the recovery room.

This was the most upsetting case I ever observed. No one, except perhaps the nurse, seemed to notice that this sixteen-year-old was shivering uncontrollably and weeping with terror. Unfortunately, a senior surgeon's lack of caring is imparted to house officers, who behaved here almost as though they were practicing veterinary medicine.[21]

Interestingly, those considered technically most gifted by their peers, such as Dr. Verdi, were frequently (although not exclusively) the most compassionate and reassuring to their patients. Such men were Exemplary Surgeons, admired by colleagues, loved by patients.

Neither untrustworthiness nor lack of caring necessarily involves surgical misbehavior. Nevertheless, each embodies a grievous moral defect. Despite the fact that they are repugnant, and profoundly disturbing, I do not classify these attributes as *deadly* surgical sins. They represent *moral* rather than *professional* misbehavior; impatience resulting in carelessness represents moral *and* professional misbehavior.

DEFICIENCIES

My fourth category of misbehavior is related neither to virtues nor to moral defects. Instead, it consists of a deficiency of attributes related to the art, craft, and science of surgery.

Ignorance and Incompetence

Neither ignorance nor incompetence merits an Aristotelian analysis. Rather than being related to a surgical virtue, both stem from an absence of the most basic characteristics necessary to become a surgeon: knowledge, judgment, and technical skill. Absent, too, are the moral virtues required to obtain knowledge and competence.[22] Both sins are inexcusable in a doctor; ignorance is culpable, incompetence murderous.

Naturally, ignorance is relative. The most poorly trained and least intelligent surgeon knows so much more than the observing anthropologist that she may have had difficulty identifying ignorance in action. Although I heard covert remarks about senior surgeons who were trained in poorly regarded overseas programs and who had difficulty in passing their specialty boards,[23] I can find no example in my field notes of unqualified ignorance displayed by a senior surgeon.

Ignorance, however, is not an all-or-nothing phenomenon: some surgeons are more intelligent, better trained, better informed than others—which means that some are less intelligent, less well trained, and less informed. Not recognizing one's *comparative* ignorance is a surgical sin. A chief of surgery remarked "God save me from the fascinating case!" He commented approvingly of another surgeon, "That man knows enough to call someone in when he can't handle something." Knowing enough to know when one doesn't know enough is difficult—especially for someone with the surgical temperament.[24] Knowing what one does *not* know requires judgment.

Almost all surgical misbehavior involves poor judgment.

This does not mean that all poor judgment involves misbehavior, nor that every example ends badly: patients can endure a good deal of poor treatment—and survive to thank the
surgeon for saving their lives.[25] Even an Exemplary Surgeon
makes mistakes. Any surgeon may select the wrong (or a less
effective) procedure, wait too long (or not long enough) to
operate, treat with the wrong (or a less effective) drug. A senior
surgeon who consistently exhibits poor judgment, however,
not knowing enough to recognize and allow for his deficiencies,[26] is a Buffoon, and is treated as such by his peers. Such a
person may be ignorant, being imperfectly trained or unable
to benefit from his training. Or he may be incompetent.

Ignorance and incompetence are frequently combined.
Thus, a surgical error caused by incompetence, when ignored,
demonstrates ignorance—and a kind of moral obtuseness:

> I was told of one man, with poor technical facility, who, during
> a colon resection, severed the superior mesenteric artery, which
> supplies blood to the colon. When a house officer complained
> that the colon was a funny color, the surgeon disregarded his
> objections, reassuring the resident that everything would be all
> right. He closed the patient, who died.

Despite the fact that he was extraordinarily caring and compassionate, this man had an abysmal reputation among his
peers. In refusing to heed the house officer's misgivings, the
surgeon exhibited not only technical incompetence, but a kind
of arrogant ignorance. Such behavior represents what Bosk
classifies as a moral as well as technical error.[27]

After eighteen months of observing operations, I found
it easier to identify blatant technical incompetence. Here are
descriptions of a young surgeon, widely characterized by his
peers as incompetent, performing two minor procedures:

> *Field Notes.* I watched Sutton [perform a breast biopsy]. He's very
> good-tempered, but he *does* seem rather klutzy. (Would I think
> so if I hadn't been told by [a colleague]? Dunno.) For example,

during the biopsy, he told the resident how the best way to take a little lump of flesh was using a needle, and stitching it, and then you can just pull it out. But, oops, the thread came out without the flesh, and they had to use clamps to grab it and then cut it out. Then, there seemed to be a third lump—they had removed two [which were sent to pathology, who telephoned their report], neither of which was malignant. [But there seemed to be] something that might be a third lump. Sutton felt it, then said to the house officer, "You don't think it's anything, do you?" [I wondered,] shouldn't he have been the one to decide? When the patient was awakened, it was the anesthesiologist who thought to say to her, "It's good news!"

✳

[During the second procedure] the lump came out in pieces; Sutton sent some to the pathologist for a frozen section and some for a "permanent biopsy." . . . It looked like chopped meat in the incision, though, where Sutton, helped by the intern, had removed the lump(s). Is that what being "rough on tissue" [a surgeon's term of opprobrium] means? . . . The pathologist called, said the frozen specimen was not a lymph node. Sutton laughed nervously and said, "Hope I got out the specimen."

Unfortunately for his patients, Sutton was not limited to minor procedures. The following notes are my reflections on an enormously complex, difficult operation performed by Sutton and a chief resident:

Field Notes. There was a feeling, to me, of disorganization throughout the operation. Everything, within the incision and in the room, seemed somehow messy and sloppy—especially within the incision. There was a feeling of no control. Carl (the chief resident) seemed more in control than Sutton. Sutton took advice from Carl—although he didn't always follow it—from the PA [physician's assistant], even from the nurses. . . . The operation reminded me, in some ways, of two little kids playing doctor with no grown-ups around to reprimand them, keep them in line, and tell them what to do if they got in trouble.

Not surprisingly, the procedure was a catastrophe; everything that could go wrong did so. Although the patient survived, he had a poor surgical result—probably less satisfactory than if he had been operated on at the university hospital, whose surgeons, Sutton told me, had tried to "steal" this case from him.

Bosk[28] discusses technical errors among house officers, resulting from imperfect skills and knowledge. Such mistakes, at the elite university hospital Bosk studied, were forgiven—but remembered. A house officer whose errors did not diminish over time was considered unsuited to surgery, and if he had not committed what Bosk defines as moral errors, was routed into another specialty.

A senior surgeon who displays ignorance and incompetence represents a failure in training or in screening. Young Dr. Sutton, for example, had finished his surgical residency two years before I observed him operate. Unlike his surgical colleagues at the health maintenance organization (HMO) where he was employed—all of whom had been educated in the Near and Far East—Sutton had attended a well-regarded American medical school. He spent his internship and part of his first year of residency at hospitals affiliated with the school, finishing his surgical training at three other, less prestigious, hospitals, and ending up at an institution that sounded rather like a rural Mount Saint Elsewhere. Why did he leave his first training program in the middle of his second year? Why did he keep moving from hospital to hospital (he received his surgical training at four hospitals)? My suspicion is that Sutton was good at being a student and poor at being a surgeon, that an ability for books and exams was matched by disabilities in technique and clinical judgment.

Bosk describes how unsuitable house officers, who were discharged by the high-ranking training program he studied, were often taken on by less prestigious hospitals.[29] Perhaps this is what happened to Dr. Sutton. Whatever the behind-the-scenes history, Sutton was graduated from a recognized training program as a qualified surgeon. He was then hired by a prepaid health plan—the only American-born, American-educated general surgeon at the HMO, and by far the least competent. I know nothing of the politics of the health plan: why Sutton was hired and why the enormously skilled, highly respected senior surgeon who supervised him kept him on, despite complaints by patients and house officers and ferocious jokes and snide remarks by colleagues. I know nothing of the politics of the community hospital where Sutton operated: why the chief of surgery, who must have been aware of his deficiencies, permitted him to perform procedures there.

I have observed house officers, widely regarded as catastrophes by peers and seniors, who were retained in training programs for understandable, but not necessarily forgivable, reasons. The fault may well be that of the chiefs of surgery who do not discharge these residents—with a reference that would make it impossible for them to be picked up by another training program.[30] The misbehavior resulting from ignorance and incompetence, however, must be placed at the surgeon's door: it is he who commits the deadly sins—and too often, they are deadly, indeed.

JUDGING SINS

The reader may wonder whether the definition and classification of surgical sins presented here is mine or that of the surgeons I studied. The behavior described here was deplored by the surgeons I studied: *they* considered it misbehavior. Although the taxonomy is my responsibility, it was inspired by surgeons' reactions to misbehavior—especially those Exemplary Surgeons whose judgment and deeds I particularly respected. The categories were influenced by what I perceive as differing responses by surgeons to different varieties of misbehavior. Such a taxonomy—refined and improved by those with a more profound knowledge of surgery—might help define appropriate reactions by surgeons and chiefs of surgery to the misbehavior of colleagues. Misbehavior is *not* a global phenomenon: one example does not have the same valence or disvalue as another. Being "against misbehavior" (the way Calvin Coolidge reported the preacher was against sin) is a weak posture, with little value for positive action.

At this point, critics may object that surgeons' reactions to misbehavior are irrelevant, that surgeons historically have colluded to ignore and justify the errors and misbehavior of colleagues (as Millman contends),[31] and that there is little reason to expect a simple classification to alter their behavior. Millman, like many critics, automatically equates mistakes with misbehavior, an approach that evokes hostility and defensiveness from doctors. If surgeons are attacked with the same ferocity for *mistakes* as for *misbehavior,* they are likely to respond by closing ranks and making strenuous efforts to conceal what goes on from outsiders. Most surgeons deplore the misbehavior of colleagues; these surgeons are in a far better position than outsiders to identify and censure such misdeeds. A classification that weights the seriousness of various kinds of misbehavior, pointing to ways for colleagues to conceptualize and cope with misdeeds, may be more effective than a punitive, regulatory approach by hostile critics.

Although vices of excess are deadly sins, and are so perceived by surgeons, they are, nevertheless, intensifications of surgical virtues. As a result, colleagues who condemn the overly heroic behavior of "gunslingers" and "matadors"[32] may covertly admire their daring and derring-do—especially when such vices produce a "miracle." Surgeons must tread a fine line between courage and recklessness, confidence and hubris, a positive attitude and a magical one. Virtues in excess are vices, to be sure, but then, a *deficiency* of surgical virtues characterizes the *wimp*—a far more derogatory attribution to someone with the surgical temperament than that of gunslinger. The connection of these vices to essential surgical attributes may help explain why surgeons have difficulty invoking harsh sanctions against colleagues who display them, feeling that "there but for the Grace of God . . . ." If the connection I posit between vices of excess and virtues is genuine, then it would be fruitless to attempt to eradicate them; all one can do is to attempt to curb them. Those who lack all susceptibility to vices of excess are probably unsuited to be surgeons.

Venality, on the other hand, can and should be criticized more readily and judged far more harshly. Although surgeons may reluctantly admire certain vices, when, for example, a gunslinger colleague produces a spectacular "save," there is little to respect in the behavior of the venal surgeon. The venal surgeon's sins generate others: his behavior is sleazy, his patients at risk. We should demand, then, that surgeons and chiefs of surgery invoke their most serious sanctions against venal colleagues. Surgeons are the most likely people to identify venality among colleagues; the proliferation of sins by a single surgeon is unmistakable to insiders. Although colleagues can claim that they were not in the operating room and consequently cannot judge what occurred—a claim frequently advanced when a colleague's errors are discussed by outsiders and one that, as we have seen, is not always true—the venal surgeon's commission of so many sins and errors contravenes the innocence and immunity claimed by colleagues. Surgeons may not want to tell the anthropologist, but they had better tell someone, and devote their most serious efforts at prohibiting venal colleagues from practicing surgery—unless they are willing to allow those critics who believe all surgeons are venal to institute the punitive and heavy-handed curbs they seek.

Venality, too, may not be an all-or-nothing phenomenon. Between Exemplary Surgeons, who never perform unnecessary or questionable procedures, and venal surgeons, who do so habitually, is a gray area—that is, unfortunately, encouraged by reimbursement patterns. Government insurance

(Medicare) that pays for almost any operation on an aged patient, an operation that the patient and the patient's family may well assent to when they do not pay the bills, encourages the "can-do" "let's-fix-it" approach common among surgeons.[33] Medicare covers simple procedures as well as complex ones: debriding (cleaning up) the bedsores of nursing-home patients, especially when performed in the operating room, where it is reimbursed at a higher rate, and doing whatever else seems indicated (or not indicated) for the nursing-home patients, can make a comfortable living for a young surgeon starting out. I have observed nursing-home patients in their nineties, clutching their stuffed teddy bears, utterly demented (permanently or temporarily), being wheeled in for an operation. I've seen others, permanently curled in a fetal position, whom some surgeons refused to operate on, enthusiastically accepted by less scrupulous colleagues. But, I have also observed patients in their sixties, seventies, and eighties, whose sufferings were diminished, capabilities enhanced, and lives prolonged through surgical intervention financed by Medicare. The reimbursement patterns of government insurance programs, such as Medicare, raise profound ethical, medical, financial, social, and legal issues that must be addressed on a society-wide basis. Until that time, however, such insurance may encourage many surgeons to perform aggressive procedures on patients whose capacity to benefit from them is questionable. (For a further discussion of some of these issues, see Chapter 8.)

Venality tends to surface when a surgeon goes into private practice. Character flaws, on the other hand, are evident in house officers, where lack of self-discipline, leading to sins such as impatience and carelessness, is judged harshly and sanctioned. Like ignorance and incompetence, we can call for even stronger sanctions against these moral flaws in a senior surgeon. It is conceivable that habitual impatience and carelessness is linked to venality. Then again, it may also be associated with a surgeon's aging ("You don't take the pains or keep going as long as perhaps you should"). The results are so deadly that we must demand that colleagues and chiefs of surgery make more serious efforts to curb those who habitually exhibit such lethal impatience—whether it results from venality, aging, or a fundamental lack of self-discipline.

Among senior surgeons, lack of self-discipline resulting in impatience and carelessness leads to poor results; untrustworthiness and lack of caring lead to unhappy patients; both generate anger, criticism, and malpractice suits. Untrustworthiness and uncaring (when they are not linked to carelessness) are frequently less severely judged than lack of self-discipline. Rather than being perceived as personal, and somewhat private characteristics, trustworthiness and caring (for the patient as a person) must consciously be imparted to surgical house officers.[34] Individual differences cannot be eradicated; some surgeons will always be more trustworthy and caring than others, just as some will be more painstaking, have better clinical judgment, or have greater technical mastery. This does not obviate the necessity to stress these characteristics—and to weed out not only house officers who do not take pains, but also those who are untrustworthy and uncaring.

I believe that those chiefs who tolerate ignorant and incompetent house officers and loose them upon the world are committing a grievous moral error. These characteristics are easily identified. Although gradations exist, Buffoons, like young Dr. Sutton, should be prevented from becoming surgeons. On occasion, a Buffoon may be one because he was poorly educated or trained. Interestingly, the same critics who attack the results of surgical ignorance and incompetence often brand sanctions against those with substandard education or training as "prejudice." This is surely a problem. So are lawsuits by discharged house officers and senior surgeons. Nevertheless, ignorant and incompetent surgeons are easily identified

by colleagues, who must be given the power—and mandate—
to punish, and if necessary, oust them, rather than washing
their hands of collegial misbehavior.

✳

In this examination of surgical misbehavior, I may have
conveyed the impression that no institutional efforts are being
made to regulate the behavior and qualifications of surgeons.
This is not so. Every hospital has a quality assurance committee, composed of doctors, that investigates complications
that occur before, during, and after surgery. Some conceal
the names of the doctors under investigation to minimize the
effects of collegiality. As far as I could tell, however, a surgeon whose complication rate was considered unacceptable
was then referred to the chief of surgery, who disposed of the
case as he saw fit. Moreover, the doctors who serve on such
committees risk being sued: in 1988, the U.S. Supreme Court
upheld an antitrust award of $2.2 million to a surgeon whose
care of patients had been criticized. The award bankrupted
some of the doctors on the committee that had sought to terminate his staff privileges at the only hospital in the town.[35]
Thus, the temptation for the small group to close ranks when
members are menaced (see page 80) is reinforced by the emotional, professional, and financial costs of disciplining collegial
misbehavior.[36]

8

IT'S NO FUN ANYMORE

My father was a lawyer. When I was a boy he often said to me, "Billy, if you're smart, when you grow up you'll be a doctor. Those bastards have it made."

William A. Nolen
The Making of a Surgeon

We had a mystique and a cult and it's gone. Today, the last thing you want to do is be introduced as a surgeon.

Thoracic surgeon

FUN AND WAR GAMES

BET YOU CAN'T do it in ten minutes!" said Dr. Villar to his partner, Dr. Desai, in the tone of one boy daring another. The patient, an eighteen-year-old booked for an emergency appendectomy, was asleep and draped on the table. Desai smiled, nodded assent, and started to open the patient, as Villar set the large OR clock to measure off the minutes. As Desai and Chuck, the intern, operated, Villar kept calling the time out: "two and a half minutes" . . . "four minutes" . . . "six and a half minutes—you'd better hurry!" The intern, who had little experience with appendixes, worked slowly and painstakingly. When he seemed to be having difficulties, Villar remarked sympathetically, "This is an operation devised by Attila the Hun!" "I'd just as soon if we went slower, OK?" responded Chuck. When Villar chanted "eight minutes," Chuck inquired nervously, "Are you going to steal this from me?" "I've got a bet!" responded Desai, but he continued talking the intern through the procedure, rather than taking over and doing it all himself. It took twenty-six minutes. I suspect Desai could have done it alone in ten.[1]

The atmosphere of bloody, boyish game playing was reminiscent of the grisly, hilarious combat stories older surgeons tell about their days as house officers: learning to give IVs with no instruction and blood spurting everywhere; crouching under the bed of an alcoholic patient, barking like a dog, so that the patient (reporting the interns' barking to the disbelieving psychiatrist) would be sent from the surgical ward to "psycho"; operating successfully after being retrieved from a surgical party (known as "liver rounds") where several drinks had been consumed, or when light-headed with fatigue, the narrator had been on call for more than forty-eight hours without sleep. Remembering similar "war" stories, related with nostalgic relish by my husband, I asked one surgeon if he had fun. "I had a ball!" he said.

The house officers I observed did not seem to be having a ball. "It's the worst year of my life!" reported an intern. The residents earned more money—despite complaints, they made enough to live on, as compared with the sixty-five to two-hundred-dollar-a-month salaries reported by the older surgeons.[2] Their hours did not seem to be quite so punishing. But the atmosphere of macabre playfulness, of gory delight in every aspect of their work, was absent. "Medicine is changing, and not for the better," reported a chief of surgery, who observed that the house officers today do not have as much of a chance to operate as he and his colleagues did, and that the young surgeons do not enjoy themselves as much. "It's less fun today," remarked the chief.

NO FUN

"Would you want your son to be a surgeon?" I asked Dr. Bryna, the Compassionate Young Surgeon (see Chapter 5). No, he would not, responded Bryna; he would not want his son to go into medicine; people have unreasonable expectations today; they assume that every problem can be taken care of and every procedure will turn out well. "It's no fun anymore," he said, and a chief resident, joining the conversation, echoed him: "It's no fun anymore!"[3]

Of seventeen men, asked if they wanted their sons or daughters to become surgeons, thirteen responded negatively. "I don't think anyone would, at this time in this climate," said one young doctor, who had spent the past year attempting, with minimal success, to support his wife and two children by the private practice of surgery. His colleague, in a similar situation, explained, "There are better ways to make money, and you could have more time with your family and more job security in another field." This theme of no fun ran like a dark undercurrent through the conversations of the surgeons I studied. Even salaried academic surgeons, freed from worries about the business of surgery, insurance premiums (covered by their employers), and the financial threats posed by malpractice suits expressed misgivings about the inimical climate of "this day and age."

The 1980s, when I conducted research, were a period of ferment in American medicine—surgery, in particular. The rules were changing—the canons of practice, procedure, relationships, and reimbursement that prevailed when this generation chose surgery—and there was no knowing what the surgery of the future would look like. "It's not a good field anymore," said one man, who told how he had "turned" his two sons and daughter "off" surgery. "You lack independence. You lack freedom."

Central to the distress of the surgeons I studied was a

sense of diminished autonomy and power. What *was* fun was
the independence celebrated in the combat narratives of older
surgeons, whose protagonists enjoyed tremendous power to
perform procedures, commit errors (if they were redeemed),
and make life-and-death decisions regarding the welfare of
patients.[4] (Their power and responsibility was, in fact, greater
than that of present house officers, for reasons that will be
discussed.

What was also fun was the conviction that one was fighting
the good war against death and disease. For the generation of
surgeons (and patients) reared during World War II, few questions existed about the necessity for battle—against invading
countries or diseases. The cause was just, the methods essential, the warrior celebrated. The underpaid and overworked
residents of the 1950s assumed without question that they
were doing good; that their efforts, however untutored and
misguided, were for the benefit of patients and humanity; and
that deference, respect, and gratitude were the natural rewards
for their exertions.

In this post-Vietnam day and age, the role of the warrior is
ill-defined and the attitude toward him ambivalent. He is re-
strained, denigrated, and at the same time, needed. War stories
from these combat zones may not reflect the same bloody delight in battle, the same conviction of the utter rightness of
one's cause, the same certainty of gratitude and support from
the home front. Although we must allow for the alchemy of
time that burnishes memories with a glow of nostalgia, re-
pressing cruelty and terror, the "old days" *were* in many respects a vanished golden age.[5]

"THE DISENCHANTMENT OF THE WORLD"

Charisma, meaning literally "gift of grace," is used by
Weber to characterize self-appointed leaders who are fol-

lowed by those who are in distress. . . . Miracles and revelations, heroic feats of valor and baffling successes are characteristic marks of their stature. Failure is their ruin.

H. H. Gerth and C. Wright Mills
"Intellectual Orientations," in
From Max Weber: Essays in Sociology

To understand the situation of surgeons "in this day and age," let us briefly consider Weber's concepts of "charisma" and its "routinization."[6] Charisma consists of "specific gifts of the body and spirit . . . believed to be supernatural, not accessible to everybody."[7] The charismatic leader exhibits his mission, or calling, by means of godlike strength or a highly personal manifestation of grace. The miracles of the prophet, the heroic deeds of the warrior-hero, demonstrate their power, which lasts only so long as their gifts can be demonstrated. The charismatic hero's mission is extinguished as soon as his followers no longer flourish.

Charisma, in this formulation, is inherently unstable, being based on very personal gifts that must be constantly demonstrated. It tends to become "routinized," giving way to rational, bureaucratic structures, governed by rules, circumscribed by regulations, administered by a cumbersome and hierarchical bureaucracy. Bureaucracy operates according to objective, "calculable" rules, without regard for persons;[8] each bureaucrat is theoretically indistinguishable from and replaceable by another with the same narrow specialization; each member of the governed is indistinguishable from and replaceable by another.

Convinced that this progression was inevitable, Weber nevertheless believed (as indicated by his reiteration of Friedrich Schiller's phrase, "the disenchantment of the world")[9] that the process exacted a high price. According to H. H. Gerth and C. Wright Mills, "Weber thus identifies bureaucracy with rationality, and the process of rationalization with mechanism, depersonalization, and oppressive routine. Rationality, in this context, is seen as adverse to personal freedom." The type of person bureaucracy selects and forms is "the narrowed professional, publicly certified and examined. . . . a petty routine creature, lacking in heroism, human spontaneity, and inventiveness." [10] Or, as the surgeon in his sixties, who lamented the loss of the mystique and cult of surgery, complained:

> Today, they're technically proficient, almost automatons; they do all these fancy procedures and act like they almost invented them—or at least charge that way! Instead of being the individualistic tough guy he used to be, today we have a swarm of technicians who come in with their lawyers and accountants and try to lock up a community. It's sort of a gray flannel suit. They don't treat patients with respect, and they think they can do more than they can. They transmit this overconfidence to the patient, which leads to lawsuits when they can't deliver.

I am arguing, then, that what surgeons find so painful in this day and age is the routinization of their charismatic authority: mechanization, depersonalization, and oppressive routines curb their freedom and autonomy; a petty bureaucratic mentality, with self-protection as its first injunction, is gradually displacing their heroic, miracle-working mystique.

First, let us examine the bureaucratic regulations that diminish the pleasure and autonomy of surgeons. Then we will explore changing attitudes toward doctors, and surgeons in particular, that erode heroism, individualism, and caring—making it difficult for anyone but a petty bureaucrat to survive.

I shall consider these processes primarily from the surgeons' point of view. (Naturally, other perspectives exist, and are pivotal in understanding the routinization of surgeons' charisma: those of laypersons—patients, families, and critics; those of members of other medical specialties, besieged by the same pressures; and of officials, concerned about the rising costs of health care.) The surgeons' outlook is the one with which I am most familiar, however, and since it is rarely expressed to laypersons, I believe it is helpful to explicate it.

THE BUREAUCRATIZATION OF CHARISMA

In the last twenty-five years, the government has instituted a series of measures to provide greater access to medical services. Government funds encouraged the expansion of hospitals, medical schools, and specialty training programs and helped financed the care of patients who were previously treated on a charity basis. Although organized medical groups fought the passage of many programs, doctors benefited financially from their initiation. To give just one example: doctors no longer had to donate all or part of their services to aged and impoverished patients; instead, they were paid on a fee-for-service basis, through Medicare and Medicaid. But, accepting these funds involved what might subsequently be defined as a Faustian bargain: doctors bought into the federal plans whose regulations they later found so oppressive.

I shall not go into the history of Medicare and Medicaid, which came into effect in 1965 to help finance medical care for the aged and the poor.[11] The regulations were, and are, complex and changing, with stringent effects upon training and practice.

The two programs had differing aims, prestige, and methods of financing. Although states differed in their provisions, a nationwide consequence of Medicaid was to curtail the number of charity (or what hospitals called "service") cases, thus diminishing the pool of patients previously cared for by young physicians in training. The cases joyfully remembered by the older surgeons from their days as house officers, when the resident "ran" the case, were now severely limited. Contemporary house officers have less responsibility for "managing" service cases. They no longer enjoy the power, independence, and autonomy celebrated in Nolen's combat stories from his days as a house officer at a public hospital in the 1950s.[12]

So far as I could determine, Medicaid had little significant financial impact upon the private practitioners I studied.

Although some might now be reimbursed for operations on "service cases" previously performed gratis, none of the practitioners I observed had practices composed primarily of such patients. (It is conceivable that Medicaid had more effect than I realized; surgeons were rather close-mouthed about their finances.) [13] Medicare, on the other hand, has had a profound effect upon surgical practice throughout the United States. The intensive care units I observed were filled with patients aged sixty-five to ninety-five years recuperating from complex and ambitious operations that would have been unheard of twenty years before.[14] Naturally, surgical techniques have evolved in the twenty-five years since Medicare was passed. But, so has the age of those upon whom these techniques are employed.

At what age and state of health does a particular procedure become an expensive luxury? Who makes the decision: the prospective patient, the patient's family, the surgeon, the state? Indicated (as surgeons would say about an operation they think appropriate) or not—and making such a decision is not simple [15]—the procedures currently performed on patients covered by Medicare are *expensive*. Almost all are paid for by taxes. And, as the costs have proliferated, so too have cost-cutting methods and measures.

From 1983 to 1986, during the period when I was studying surgeons, the government instituted a series of regulations designed to cut Medicare costs and monitor quality. These were complex.[16] Different measures were initiated at different times in different states. Different bureaucratic entities were put in charge of these measures. One week, an announcement concerning a new regulation would be made at a weekly surgeons' meeting I attended; the following week, the information might be revised or contradicted. Some regulations, pertaining to hospitals, affected surgeons (and other doctors) only indirectly. Others concerned surgeons directly, listing particular procedures that would not be reimbursed unless specific guidelines were followed: various procedures were "disallowed" unless a second opinion, from another surgeon, supporting the necessity for the operation, was obtained; then, at a later date, second opinions were discouraged, since they proved more, rather than less, expensive. To be reimbursed for certain operations, such as removing a gallbladder, surgeons had to telephone a monitoring organization and receive permission ahead of time from the nurse staffing the phone. Emergency operations performed without permission had to be retrospectively approved. Some operations were no longer reimbursed unless they were performed on an "ambulatory" basis—with the patient arriving at the hospital the day of the operation and leaving after the procedure. The requirements were complex and constantly changing. All involved time, trouble, and vast amounts of paperwork.[17] Theoretical categories—based on statistical averages and administered by bureaucratic entities—governed concrete decisions involving flesh-and-blood patients. Patients were treated as diseases rather than persons; the patient was "a gallbladder," or a "hip replacement," not an individual with a unique history, physiology, and needs.

One might argue, as indeed some did, that surgeons had exploited Medicare, that they had performed procedures on aged patients that would never have been attempted before the age of automatic reimbursement; and that now, they could cut back on the scope and number of procedures on Medicare patients, or alternatively, comply with the regulations stimulated by their greed. This punitive approach is, however, somewhat simplistic. Medicare encouraged the expectations of *patients* as well as surgeons: patients and surgeons became habituated to seeking surgical solutions to the problems of aging and the associated burden of disease. New medical and surgical developments, combined with subsidized care, made health in one's later years appear less a dream or a hope, and more a *right*. This was not necessarily a question of greed— on the part of patients or surgeons. Many surgeons quite honestly believed that their procedures could help older patients, and the operations they performed frequently did improve the quality of life and even prolong the lives of patients over the age of sixty-five.

Unfortunately, bureaucratic solutions to human problems often generate new problems. Regulations designed to cut costs and curtail unnecessary operations were circumvented with ease by dishonest surgeons. The sleazier the surgeon, the less trouble he had slithering through the complex requirements; he simply lied about what he had done, was doing, and intended to do. Instead, it was the surgeons who honestly attempted to comply with the regulations who had difficulties, since the means of compliance were unclear, the time requirements taxing, and the effect on patients frequently inimical.[18] It was the patient's *disease category*, rather than that particular patient's medical, social, and psychic needs that dictated the treatment: which tests should be performed and which, omitted, as statistically unrewarding; whether or not the patient should be hospitalized; and how long the hospitalization should extend. A surgeon who cared about a patient's welfare was frequently forced to "go around" the regulations to obtain what he believed to be proper care for that patient.[19] Thus, rather than curbing the excesses of dishonest surgeons, many of the "regs" turned relatively honest surgeons into liars.

"Going around the regs" did not only benefit patients. As surgeons often pointed out to me with some bitterness, if in complying with the regulations, a patient's welfare was jeopardized, *they* were the ones who were legally liable for the consequences.

Regulations designed to limit the costs of Medicare had a ripple effect. "First the feds, then the blues" predicted a chief of surgery in ominous tones. Versions of the federal regulations were being adopted by Blue Cross/Blue Shield ("the blues"), and other medical insurance plans were following suit. Few patients in the United States today pay for all of their medical care out of pocket. The indigent who are ineligible for Medicaid pay little or nothing; the poor and aged are covered by Medicaid and Medicare; the remainder are covered by some variety of private medical (or "third-party") insurance. The private plans were as interested in cutting costs as the federal government, and surgeons darkly predicted a day in the not-too-distant future when their practice and fees would be "totally regulated." As far as the surgeons could anticipate, the future guidelines, like the regulations initiated by the "feds," would limit surgical fees and limit the number of days patients might be hospitalized for particular diseases—but would place no limit on surgeons' legal liability.

From the surgeons' viewpoint, this would be the worst of all possible worlds. "Total regulation" would combine the financial disadvantages to doctors of socialized medicine with, as they saw it, its medical disadvantages to patients, while omitting the legal advantages of socialized plans, where doctors are employed, reimbursed, and protected by the state. The feds and third-party insurers would make the decisions; the surgeons could be sued for the consequences.

THE EROSION OF CHARISMA

Something else was occurring in the 1980s that was even more painful and puzzling to surgeons than "the regs": people's attitudes toward doctors were undergoing profound and inimical changes.

When I asked a full-time academic surgeon if he would want his son to be a surgeon, he responded, "No, not even a doctor!" explaining: "What made me go into medicine in the first place is not there anymore. Society changed in its attitude toward physicians. I went in not for the lure of making a lot of money but for what I perceived my role would be. I would make all these sacrifices, but I would be someone special, and people's looks would tell me that." Expectations about medicine have not changed, he affirmed, just attitudes toward doctors. He said: "People want just as much, if not more, from medicine, but they don't think so much of doctors anymore. . . . At any gathering, someone puts down doctors. It's as if you paid money and bought the doctor—not just *his services*, but *the doctor.*"

A chief resident expressed similar sentiments. As he got educated, people always said things would be harder, he observed. And yes, first grade was harder than kindergarten; and medical school was even harder than people told him it would be; and being a house officer is hard; and he doesn't get enough money—residents make less than the nurses— but that doesn't bother him. What bothers him is that surgeons don't get the respect they used to get. They still do, in some parts of the country, he reported, but in urban situations there's no respect: people just want to sue and get all the money they can. He doesn't mind working hard, and he doesn't mind not being rich, he complained, but he really feels strongly about the change in attitude toward doctors.

Critical books, articles, and news features about doctors have combined anger and expectation. Those critics who excoriated the venality, stupidity, and greed of doctors expressed rage that the arts of these presumably venal, stupid, and greedy doctors were not infallible. The newspaper columns debunking last year's miracles, showing how they were based upon imperfect evidence and false assumptions, were followed by panegyrics to new medical and surgical techniques. The social scientists who belittled surgeons as a greedy, overpaid, arrogant crew, revered their own surgeons, confidently expecting them to produce miracles when required.

Weber observed that "the charismatic leader gains and maintains authority solely by proving his strength in life. If he wants to be a prophet, he must perform miracles. . . . Above all, however, his divine mission must 'prove' itself in that those who faithfully surrender to him must fare well. If they do not fare well, he is obviously not the master sent by the gods."[20] Because their miracles could not be relied upon, surgeons as a group were losing their charismatic authority. The *hope* for miraculous cures had been transformed into *expectation;* when a technique or treatment failed, patients and their families reacted not with disappointment but *blame.* Critics, commentators, and laypersons seemed to make an automatic, unspoken assumption: that medical and surgical failure derived from error; that errors were equivalent to misbehavior; and that such misbehavior comprised malpractice.

Patients and families became more demanding—and accusatory: "There is no such thing as an easy family anymore!" as one surgeon remarked to a colleague (see page 52).

Middle-class patients were, perhaps, the most difficult. They had read the articles, the news features—even the medical journals. Rejecting the traditional hierarchical relationship between doctor and patient, they wanted to share in their medical care, to be, so far as possible, partners in decision making.[21] Such a partnership rejects the charismatic leader-follower relationship; rather than "surrendering" to the prophet-healer's powers, the patient seeks agency, alliance, parity. Such "egalitarian" decision making requires an enormous investment of time and psychic energy from doctors.

An internist described two patients with breast cancer who were giving him "a terrible time." They have to know about *everything,* he said. They're so distrustful; they have to manage everything. One patient's husband insisted upon seeing the operative note dictated by her surgeon. The internist reported that a surgical colleague, who sat in on one of these conferences, couldn't believe what was going on. He had to warn the surgeon to keep his patience. "It takes longer if you get exasperated," the internist cautioned. The surgeon subsequently expressed nostalgia for the good old days of his surgeon father, who would announce to the patient what was wrong, what he intended to do, and what the procedure would cost.

Not every doctor has the patience, interpersonal sensitivity—and time—to meet the demands of distrustful middle-class patients who insist on knowing everything and managing every detail. Such time is emotionally and financially costly.

And yet, those patients who demand empathetic, time-consuming, individual care from their doctors are frequently those who wish to reduce the price of that care. Those patients who demand intensely *personal* care are frequently those who depersonalize their doctors, acting as though their "health-care providers" were interchangeable cogs. "Cut the Cost, Keep the Care" proclaimed a 1984 advertisement by the American Association of Retired Persons. The contradictions embodied by such demands are more apparent to doctors than to patients.

A young surgeon predicted: "It's going to end up like Mountain View Group Health [a prepaid health plan]; that's the wave of the future, with surgeons like Sutton [the hospital Buffoon; see pages 173–76]. People will get what they think they want!" Practitioners were convinced that the salaried surgeon of the future—with his eight-hour day, five-day week, and prescheduled time slots for each patient—would have less personal involvement with patients. Cutting costs, working hours, and patient time would diminish commitment, and consequently, the quality of care. The charismatic hero would be replaced by the "health-care provider," a petty bureaucrat, interchangeable with all others like him, who treated patients as interchangeable cogs. An Exemplary Surgeon, who advised his daughter to go into anesthesiology ("no trouble, no grief, good hours, the patient doesn't bother you"), anticipated that surgical patients would not get the same kind of care in the salaried future. "But then, they don't want it," he declared.

Lamenting the depersonalization, the diminished respect, autonomy, and financial promise of "this day and age," a surgeon in his forties said:

> We're gonna be the first generation, my generation of physicians, who are *not* going to encourage their children into medicine. . . . I always looked forward, you know, like when I first started private practice, that Rick [his partner] and I would be turning over the practice to his sons and my son and my daughter, you know, a family practice. But now, I don't know. Everybody's considering me a vendor, or I'm a provider; I'm a vendor, and this is a consumer—they took away the integrity! Now, they're even taking away the money. For fifteen years of education and torture, working 120 hours a week, and getting aggravated, and losing a lot of sleep, even in private practice. It's not worth it. . . . No one trusts us. There's no integrity.

The diminishing prestige and authority of doctors is reflected in the aspirations and behavior of nurses. Today's nurse aspires to be an independent professional, rather than simply "the handmaiden of the doctor." No longer content with being a subordinate member of the team, nurses cast themselves as "the patient's advocate," protecting patients from doctors' mistakes and misbehavior. Feminist critiques point out that the division of labor in the operating room, for example, where male doctors take active, decision making positions and female nurses are confined to supportive and childlike roles, is neither necessary nor "natural."[22] During the course of research, I did, indeed, observe OR nurses being treated like children; at the same time, however, I observed many OR nurses behave in a rather literal and childlike fashion. I cannot tell whether the treatment or the behavior came first; it is conceivable that those who seek more independence and autonomy leave nursing, or move to subspecialties where they are given more responsibility.[23] Whatever the justification, an angry and resentful OR nurse aggravates the surgeon's complex and demanding task: when he extends his palm, he wants the correct instrument placed in it—not a question, comment, or critique. Surgeons are convinced that in the operating room, as in war, hierarchy is essential, that orders must be followed promptly and unquestioningly if one is to win the battle against disease and death. Like patients, however, today's nurses want to be treated as allies, not subordinates.

Although the resentment, distrust, and demands are directed at *all* doctors, I believe that surgeons suffer disproportionately from their impact. The reasons are symbolic, temperamental, and historical.

Surgery is the specialty that implicitly promises the miraculous cures patients seek; and, in return for their capacity to work miracles, surgeons have enjoyed unparalleled prestige, respect, and affluence. Their arrogance, egotism, and decisiveness can be reassuring when these attributes result in miracles, and infuriating when no miracles are forthcoming. Dostoyevski's Grand Inquisitor (in *The Brothers Karamazov*) argues that freedom is too dangerous and frightening for weak, fallible humans, that people must have "miracle, mystery, and authority." The surgeon, more than any other medical specialist, represents charismatic miracle, mystery, authority— forces that are longed for, feared, resented. The surgeon, then, symbolizes the hopes, fears, and disappointments of today's patients, tempted by reports of medical miracles, terrified by disorder and disease, enraged at the invisible, unknowable forces that made them ill.

In addition, the surgeon, more than other medical specialists, represents the seductive, terrifying world of technology. Anthropologist Robert Redfield contrasts *the moral order,*" the binding together of men through implicit convictions as to what is right," with *the technical order,* organized by necessity or expediency, where "men are bound by things, or are themselves things." [24] Surgeons, who present themselves as technicians and are, in many ways, a species of glorified technician (see page 30), may symbolically represent this technical order, which lacks the human connection, conscience, and caring of the moral order. Technology is cold and inhuman (an accusation leveled against surgeons); its inappropriate and uncritical use can cause suffering, rather than cure. People's ambivalence toward the promise and threat of technology, which can save lives at the same time as it transforms people into objects, is expressed in their attitudes toward surgeons.

In temperament and attitude, surgeons are less equipped than members of other specialties to meet the moral and emotional demands of contemporary patients: to talk with (not *to*) them; to share decision making; to comfort and keep them company as they descend into the valley of the shadow of death. The daring, arrogance, decisiveness, and *machismo* that characterize surgeons rarely coexist with the gentleness, empathy, and compassion today's patients call for; the hierarchy of charismatic authority ill accords with the sharing of responsibility middle-class patients seek.

Traditionally, the surgeon was free to exercise absolute power; he could cast himself as king of the operating room, tyrant of the consulting chamber. A family story illustrates the despotism of the Old-Time Prima Donna. "During the 1930s my grandmother saw a specialist about a melanoma on her face. During the course of the visit when she asked him a question, he slapped her face, saying, 'I ask the questions here. I'll do the talking!'"[25]

Such arrogance and insensitivity is no longer tolerated—by patients, chiefs of surgery, or hospital administrators. The change is unquestionably beneficial for patients. Nevertheless, even surgeons who are warm, caring, and compassionate may regret their loss of power and authority. "Surgery is not the same as the old days," said an Exemplary Surgeon in his late fifties. "Today, when I'm ready to do a breast procedure, I have to explain all sorts of things." (I had the impression he felt some of these things were not necessarily good for the patient to hear or decide about.) "Of course," he added hastily, "it may be better for the patient, but it's not as much fun," he said regretfully. "There's not the same personal involvement—sometimes I think I'd like to retire and just do hernias." Another surgeon, a longtime personal friend, was even more open: "I was trained to tell people what was best for them," he said, "to make the decision and then just *tell* them. Perhaps the new way is better for the patient, and surely it's more democratic, but I find it *hard*," he complained. "It's not how I learned to do things."

People expect more from their surgeons, then, and get angrier at them when they do not deliver. At the same time, surgeons are probably less able than members of other specialties to meet many of the social and emotional demands of today's patients. The flip side of the surgeon as culture hero,[26] whom patients revere and obey, is the surgeon as villain, whom patients blame—and sue.

HORROR STORIES: THE PATIENT AS ENEMY

A general surgeon related the following story:

> He was in the emergency room when a seventeen-year-old boy was brought in. Playing Russian roulette with friends (inspired by the then-popular film, *The Deer Hunter*), the boy had shot himself in the head with a Vietnam veteran father's revolver. The bullet had entered the right temple, exiting at the top of his skull, blowing off much of the right side of his head (a CAT scan showed extensive intracranial injury). The boy suffered a respiratory arrest in the ER and was saved by the narrator. He then was operated on twice by a neurosurgeon to debride (cleanse) the brain tissue. After being transferred from the intensive care unit to the surgical ward, the patient tried to get out of bed without help and slid down to the floor. (X rays revealed that he did not hit his head at this time, said the surgeon.) After a number of additional neurosurgical operations, the boy returned home and did fairly well, managing to graduate from high school and lead a relatively

normal life. After the final operation, when a metal plate was put in the boy's head to cover the defect, the family sued the neurosurgeon and the hospital, contending that it was the boy's sliding out of bed that had necessitated all the subsequent operations.

Over the years, I have heard innumerable stories of this genre: some describe firsthand experience; some concern friends and acquaintances; some involve almost mythical, unnamed characters. The account can be classified as a doctor-patient "horror story,"[27] a description of what can go wrong in the relationship between doctors and patients.

These narratives come in two main varieties: doctors' stories and patients' stories. Doctors' horror stories depict patients as exploitive, demanding, and predatory; patients' horror stories depict doctors as negligent, venal, and uncaring. Each have credibility—when they concern firsthand experience. Despite their possible veracity, what such narratives signify is complex. Rather than recounting customary, average, or statistically meaningful occurrences, the stories are cautionary: they describe what *might* happen, what *on rare occasion* actually does happen, what doctors and patients *fear* will happen.[28] It is not the statistical incidence of such events that make doctor-patient horror stories pivotal, but the climate of anxiety and distrust they document—and augment. Like the perennial description of the razor blade in the Halloween apple, the horror stories are a kind of contemporary folklore or mythology; they exemplify people's fears and affect their behavior.

Patients' stories are widely circulated. Everyone knows someone who knows someone to whom something horrifying was done by a doctor.[29] Doctors encounter patients' stories in newspapers, on television, from "friends" and strangers. As the surgeon remarked, "The last thing you want to do is be introduced as a surgeon." When you are so introduced, someone is only too eager to relate several horror stories.

Patients' stories concern psychic, technical, or financial misbehavior. Interestingly, I do not recall hearing patients' horror stories about occurrences that resulted in lawsuits,[30] although the narrators seem to assume, without question, that the misbehavior they describe constitutes a variety of malpractice. In similar fashion, laypersons take it for granted that every malpractice suit they hear about involves misbehavior.

Perhaps one reason even relatively sophisticated laypersons assume the equivalence between malpractice suits and misbehavior is that they do not hear the doctor-patient horror stories doctors tell. Such stories generally involve malpractice suits or threats to sue. Not surprisingly, they concern actions that by no stretch of the imagination could be equated with misbehavior—this is what makes them *horror* stories.

I shall concentrate here on surgeons' stories. This is, of course, one-sided: patients' stories are equally valid, equally horrifying—in some ways, more horrifying, since patients have less power than the doctors who mistreat them. Patients' stories, however, are more widely circulated than those of doctors. In this study of surgeons, I want to explore *their* perceptions of what they simply call "malpractice"; this term refers to patients' lawsuits, threats of such suits, and the financial and psychic costs of these threats. Surgeons' perceptions of "malpractice" are omnipresent: when they consult with patients, operate, make rounds, and discuss cases.[31]

Let us consider another horror story told by a surgeon in 1985, concerning a malpractice suit that had been settled a few days earlier:

> In 1973, a man was brought to the emergency room suffering from an aneurysm (a ballooning of a weakened part of an artery which can be fatal if it "blows"). After an hour in the ER, he was taken to the operating room. On the table, the patient suffered a cardiac arrest before the narrator began to operate; the surgical team resuscitated him and repaired the aneurysm. After the operation, the patient had an infarct and died. The family sued the hospital, the internist, and the surgeon. They really had no case, said the surgeon; the patient had suffered an earlier infarct in the emergency room before being operated on. The suit "hung

over his head" for twelve years. Three days before it came to trial, the surgeon's lawyer (retained by his insurance company) telephoned and said the family was willing to settle: the hospital had agreed to give them $250,000; the internist had agreed to give them $150,000; and all he had to do was to agree to give them $150,000 as well (which his insurance would cover). "No way!" said the surgeon. "Bring it to trial, I'm not going to settle!" The day of the suit, his lawyer telephoned and said the family had dropped him from the charge. This means, explained the surgeon, that they got all that money—and if he had caved in, they would have gotten $150,000 more.

First, let me note that the narrator was an Exemplary Surgeon, respected by colleagues, juniors, and members of the community where he practiced. The suit was unjustified: the patient had almost died before being operated on, and would surely have died without medical care.[32] The patient died because of an aneurysm, not malpractice. His death did not derive from "failure to exercise the degree of reasonable and ordinary care, diligence, and skill in the diagnosis and treatment of his patient that physicians engaged in the same line of practice during the same period of time ordinarily possess and exercise."[33]

Why did the family sue? Did they need money, now that their husband and father—a relatively young man—was dead? Did they conclude that the doctors and hospitals were insured and "it would not cost them"? In this respect, another story is illustrative:

A universally admired and beloved chief of surgery closed a patient after operating on him, leaving a sponge behind; the nurses had counted incorrectly, and the chief did not know a sponge was missing. The team had to reoperate and retrieve the sponge. The patient sued and, quite naturally, the chief lost: there was nothing to say; it was his responsibility. A year later, when the same man needed another operation, he came to the chief, who was astounded. "I knew it wasn't your fault, Doc," said the patient. "I wouldn't let anyone else operate on me!"

For some patients and families, their feelings about their doctor, his competence, caring, and probity, are irrelevant: business is business.

Another reason why the family whose husband and father died from an aneurysm sued suggests itself: perhaps they sued because they had an overwhelming need to blame someone, anyone, for the terrible tragedy that befell them.

When E. E. Evans-Pritchard studied an African people, the Azande, in the 1920s, he noted that although the Azande understand causality as do we, unlike us, they attribute serious misfortune—especially if it results in death—to the actions of a witch.[34] If, for example, an old wooden granary happened to collapse on a group of people and kill them, the Azande would understand how termites could eat away the supports of a wooden building, and how people might be sitting under that building to avoid the midday sun; nevertheless, they would attribute the coincidence of the two happenings to witchcraft. The tragedy would be the *fault* of a witch (whose identity could be discovered by means of a poison oracle). The anthropologist's comparisons between the Azande, who believe in witchcraft, and "we," who do not, are less engaging today than in the 1930s, when they were first published. The beliefs and behavior of American patients in the 1980s resemble, in many respects, those Evans-Pritchard described for the Azande. Patients and families do not attribute serious misfortune—especially if it results in death—to God's will, fate, or statistical chance. Someone must be *at fault*. To quote the Azande: "Death always has a cause, and no man dies without a reason."

Not only patients, but juries, affix blame for misfortune. As a chief of surgery said to a group of medical students, "The insurance system is changing from a·system for punishing an outstanding wrongdoer to one for rewarding patients whom something has happened to."[35]

Why don't more doctors react like the surgeon who de-

clared, "Bring it to trial. I'm not going to settle!" Why did the
hospital and internist give in, if they were convinced that they
were not at fault? Critics assume that it is knowledge of their
own culpability that makes doctors and hospitals settle suits
before they go to trial. Such critics disregard the time and psychic energy it takes to fight a malpractice charge. Persuaded
that juries award money on the basis of sympathy, rather than
malfeasance, few doctors have the strength, conviction—and
just plain guts—to see a case through. (The reactions of this
particular surgeon illustrate some of the characteristics that
render him Exemplary.) Still fewer doctors will refuse to settle
a second time, after undergoing the shocking and humiliating
experience of losing a malpractice suit when they are certain
that no negligence occurred.

   With what they perceive as biased juries, grasping and
heartrending defendants, aggressive lawyers for the plaintiffs,
and what they believe to be inadequate defense lawyers,[36]
many surgeons feel as though whatever they do can and will
be misconstrued:

> During an operation, a urologist was deciding whether to remove
> all or part of a patient's testicle after a suspicious hard spot was
> discovered. "You get sued fifty percent of the time, anyhow," he
> declared. "If it's malignant and you don't remove it you get sued;
> if you remove it and it *isn't* malignant, you get sued." He said he
> had a suit pending against him for five million dollars. He had
> observed a patient for six months to determine whether or not
> the man had a malignancy; the patient consulted a competitor,
> who removed the testicle; it was the right time to do it, and the
> testicle turned out to be malignant. His insurance company con-
> tacted him, saying, "You have only three million dollars' worth
> of insurance; do you have any more with someone else?"

Again:

> Two surgeons discussed whether a patient should be moved to
> get a CAT scan; she was having difficulties after an operation, and

her surgeon wanted documentation in case of a suit. The patient's condition was not stable, however, and she could not be moved without danger. Later, the second surgeon said that his colleague would be in trouble if the patient's lawyer declared, "So you didn't rule out [a possible complication] with a CAT scan, Doctor?"; but he would also be in trouble if the lawyer inquired, "So you moved a patient who wasn't stable just to do a test, Doctor?" "Catch-22!" remarked the surgeon.

Even an unjustified suit, one that vindicates the surgeon, can be a burden. The most sensitive, conscientious, and caring people may be those who feel such pressures most intensely. A friend related the following story:

An accident victim was brought into an emergency room with a back injury; he was seen there by the ER doctor. The staff, who transferred the patient from the stretcher to a litter to take him to radiology to be x-rayed, neglected to stabilize his head. The patient's neck was fractured, and he was paralyzed. An orthopedist and a neurosurgeon were called in; both declared that the paralysis was irreversible. No one was able to determine whether it was due to the original accident or the move from the stretcher. The patient sued everyone connected with the case, including the orthopedist, who was not in the hospital when the patient was moved. During the ten years the case took to come to trial, the orthopedist was so upset that he sought psychiatric counseling. After the suit was settled—he was exonerated—the orthopedist retired, several years earlier than planned. "I don't have to subject myself to this!" he said.

I have discussed the "paranoia" of surgeons (pages 50–58), who feel "everyone's against them, even disease." Not surprisingly, malpractice threats heighten such paranoia. The ten or twelve years until a suit comes to trial is a long time to wait and wonder and worry, especially if the surgeon is protected by one million dollars' worth of insurance against a suit for five million. "They're going after personal assets!" announced a chief of surgery in 1985; whether or not this and similar reports were factual, surgeons believed them and exchanged grim accounts of colleagues being stripped of worldly goods. "Many of us are thinking of giving our assets to our wives," said one man, "so if we get sued they couldn't take everything." Their house was in his wife's name, he asserted, but he worried about his retirement money. Another contended that surgeons should cancel their insurance, that "the lawyers won't go after you if you have no money." He contemplated banking his earnings in Switzerland after declaring them and paying taxes, and turning over whatever he had in the United States to his wife and children. "I think about moving elsewhere," he said, "but I don't think I really will."

Among the stories surgeons exchanged was one about a gynecologist who had recently won the state lottery and soon afterwards had four lawsuits pending against her. "Everyone thinks she's rich, and they want theirs," explained the narrator, who continued, "The funny thing is that her husband, a urologist, bought the tickets, but he used her name because he didn't want these troubles himself, if he won!"

Surgeons acted as though the voice of the prosecuting attorney constantly echoed in their consciousness. While operating or discussing cases, one would often break into hectoring mimicry.

> During an operation, a resident in general surgery told how he had been assisting gynecologists with hysterectomies so that when he went into private practice he could do his own. "You can't do that!" said a senior surgeon, taking an aggressive, theatrical tone and inquiring: "How many hysterectomies have you done in the past year, Doctor? Is this a routine procedure with you?" Another senior surgeon joined in, with additional mock-malpractice-trial questions. Explanation was unnecessary; everyone understood the exchange.

I observed surgeons taking three samples for testing, rather than one, explaining that, if a lawyer asked, they could not be faulted for doing only one test, which might be inaccurate, or even only two, which might be unreliable. When a patient was transferred from one hospital to another, the second surgeon took X-rays (even though the patient arrived with a complete set). He explained that a colleague had lost a suit because he could not document a patient's condition when the man was removed from the ambulance. Practicing this kind of defensive medicine was less fun, said many.

Those who insist that doctors "Cut the Cost, Keep the Care" are likely to be the critical, vocal, and aware "consumers" who sue if a retrospectively necessary test was not performed. They want to dispense with *unnecessary* tests. But, since tests are ordered on the statistical probability that they will determine something of importance, the more tests, the higher the probability that nothing will be overlooked. Naturally, the higher the costs, as well. Before the "age of malpractice," the cutoff point for tests was some kind of balancing between the probability of determining something significant and the costs to patients. But, when the probability of being sued is added to the probability that tests will determine something about the patient's condition, the result is proliferating tests and escalating costs.

Performing expensive and relatively unnecessary tests is only one kind of defensive medicine. Another is the "turfing" of complex, challenging cases to university hospitals where patients will be cared for by famous surgeons who (so practitioners believe) are less vulnerable to suits.

> A surgeon at a community hospital told of a local politician with a son who had cancer. He sent the boy to a distant university hospital, where his leg was amputated at the hip. The boy died a year later. The same thing would have happened if *he* had operated, declared the surgeon, but the family would have been far more likely to blame him for the results.

In an OR lounge, I heard an older man counsel a younger colleague: "With the high malpractice today, people don't want to do difficult complicated cases; they send them away. Just do bread-and-butter cases and don't expose yourself to risk. Why run the risk of a malpractice suit?"

Not only difficult *cases*, but difficult *patients*, may be shunned. Many doctors believe that patients who complain, demand, threaten, or refuse to follow orders are those who subsequently sue. Describing the kind of patient he avoids, one man explained, "For example, people who come to you and say how they've been screwed up by their previous doctor; they'll usually end up saying that about you." Patients who have already initiated a suit against a doctor have demonstrated what they do when they are dissatisfied. "Why run the risk of a malpractice suit?" as the surgeon advised.

Naturally, it's less fun for a surgeon to avoid challenges, to ring himself round with defensive tests and X rays, to spend more precautions on avoiding suits than on making patients better. The better, braver, more daring surgeons, then, may be more vulnerable to suits than those prudent souls who spend much of their time and energy following the cardinal rule for the man in the gray flannel suit: *cover your ass.*

The necessity to protect oneself against the omnipresent threat of lawsuits is alienating. It's difficult not to feel somewhat distant and antagonistic toward someone you know may turn on you at any time. Although one may care *for* patients, caring *about* them may become harder. Recall the words of the young surgeon, who believed that caring about patients made them better faster:

> Caring about a patient means inquiring about them several times a day, seeing them several times a day. I think seeing a patient several times a day because you care about them can pick up the fact that the NG [nasogastric] tube is not draining well, that it needs to be irrigated; and just by accident, you'll have been in there because you care about the patient, you can fix the NG tube and make it work.

Such caring, such conscientiousness, such concentration of effort and attention involves something close to love. This gift cannot be purchased, demanded, extorted. It is bestowed freely, or not at all.

But it is difficult to give oneself freely to someone poised to sue. When the doctor is perceived as a potential antagonist, the patient too becomes an enemy.

9

EXPECTED MIRACLES

To continue to blame biomedicine exclusively for its ills is to reproduce its own ideology—that it is independent of society and has an exclusive relationship with nature. Biomedicine's practices take place against a particular background of what it means to be human. When calling it "dehumanizing" we do well to consider what it means in western society to be "human."

Deborah R. Gordon
"Tenacious Assumptions in Western
Medicine," in *Biomedicine Examined*

Today, the essentially social doctor/patient relationship is undergoing an even more intense socialization. Patients, who since the earliest times have thought of medical care as a benefit, now consider it a right and one automatically enjoyed by everyone. The very appearance of illness, instead of being considered a misfortune, becomes for some, a violation of a "right to health" for which compensation is owed.

James F. Drane
*Becoming a Good Doctor: The Place of
Virtue and Character in Medical Ethics*

WHAT OF PATIENTS?

*T*HIS BOOK has a crucial omission. In it, I explore the world of surgeons from their perspective, indicating how they perceive their work, colleagues, and communities. But I pay little attention to patients, except as bearers of disease to be meliorated or cured by surgeons' procedures, or as adversaries, bent upon avenging their thwarted desire for miracles.

I am aware that patients are at the center of the medical enterprise. I am also aware that for surgeons, however compassionate, every patient is one of many, while for patients, however ill, every operation is unique.

Let us reverse our focus and briefly examine the relationship between surgeons and patients from the patient's perspective.[1] This is, after all, my own outlook. I, too, fear illness. I, too, worry at 2:00 A.M. about what will happen if I get sick, about how to find a competent and compassionate doctor, about how my doctors will care for me and whether they will care *about* me.

All of us, including doctors, have been or will be patients. Many, including doctors, have been or will be subjected to the "sharp compassion" of the surgeon's art. All of us will be lonely, frightened, hopeful, furious at the twist of fate that extricated us from the immediacy and dailiness of our lives to thrust us into "the kingdom of the sick."[2] We will all suffer profoundly: from our ailments, our fears, the need for fateful decisions, the torments and uncertainties of treatments and tests, and from the effects of surgery itself. We will have need of tenderness and compassion as much as cure—more, if our ailments prove to be chronic, unresectable, incurable.

When cure is achieved, our suffering appears justified: it can be factored as one of the costs of the surgical miracle. Although cure does not erase suffering, it allows us to return to our everyday reality and attempt to forget the pain, terror, and disorder of the kingdom of the sick. Each of us can begin to reconstitute our shattered sense of self, of intactness, of invulnerability.

Even when we have been cured, however, the price seems, somehow, excessive. Why do so many feel we were given so little information, support, reassurance, loving care, and consideration from the men (and most frequently, they were men) in whose hands we put our lives? Many of us were cured. But were we healed?

When our sufferings did not elicit a miracle, when we were neither cured nor healed, we may well react with fury and frustration. We paid a grievous price, in pain, fear, and blasted hopes, and were repaid in false coin. How dare our surgeon retreat behind a shield of objectivity, hiding behind the mask of mere mechanic or technician, when we entrusted him with our lives, our fate? How dare he not be moved by our suffering, how dare he not show sorrow and compassion for our state?

Who then will help patients? Who will comfort us and accompany us through the medical labyrinth to meet the terrible secret at its heart?

Alas, few surgeons are as gifted at easing dread, disorder, unwellness as they are at excising diseased tissue. Few have the same ability to mitigate suffering as they do to cure disease. Just as the surgical miracle has limits, surgeons, too, have their limits. Although many may care *about* as well as *for* their patients, and some may have the ability to heal as well as cure, Exemplary Surgeons are rare. Surgeons, in the final reckoning, must be judged by their technical gifts—without these, they are charlatans; but when surgeons possess technique, knowledge, and clinical judgment, they may also be cold and uncaring, while being effective at curing disease.

Rather than reacting with anger and blame, raging because all surgeons are not exemplary, lamenting because they lack the temperament and ethos of, say, pediatricians or psychiatrists, perhaps we must begin to design structural arrangements that assure patients the caring, compassion, and comfort they require. Blaming surgeons for what they are *not* is futile. Naturally, we must encourage training that stresses the importance of caring: that teaches surgeons how to *visit*, rather than making rounds; how to talk with patients carefully and caringly; how to recognize fear and know how to allay it. We must recognize, however, that the kind of person who goes into surgery may not be notable for gentleness, empathy, and compassion. Trying to alter surgeons' temperament and ethos is more difficult and fruitless than augmenting the areas where they are likely to be lacking.[3]

Once we acknowledge the gulf between most surgeons' abilities and almost all patients' needs, we can stop ridiculing, deploring, denouncing, and begin to *understand* what is going on. Only when we understand a problem can we address ourselves to its solution.

EXPECTING MIRACLES

The title of this book, *Expected Miracles*, is of course an oxymoron, a contradiction in terms. The essence of miracles (as their linguistic derivation from the Latin verb *mira*, "to wonder at," suggests) is their uniqueness, mystery, and unexpectedness. Were these happenings utterly routine and predictable, they would not be miracles.

In discussing the surgical "miracle," I have noted that my use of the term is metaphorical. Surgical cures do not derive from the healing touch of a being endowed with supernatural abilities. Nevertheless, in some respects they resemble miracles. To repeat my argument: like miracles, successful operations are rapid, spectacular, definitive, and attributable; they are performed by someone with remarkable powers; they have an aspect of mystery and unpredictability.

Surgical miracles, however, have their limits. Today, a growing number of patients suffer from chronic illnesses for which no cure is known.[4] The surgeon's efforts may palliate symptoms or postpone death, but they cannot restore a chronic patient to health.

Moreover, even in situations where "miracles" may be achieved, their occurrence cannot be taken for granted. Although the statistical incidence of success may be known—for a particular operation on someone with a particular disease— *each time that operation is to be performed on a specific patient, the result cannot unequivocally be known in advance.* Chance is an integral part of the surgeon's universe. Patients may hope for cure, pray for cure, but they cannot *depend* upon being cured by the surgeon's art. The same indifferent fate that determines one's disease affects one's cure.

This is bitter knowledge, indeed.

The relationship between surgeon and patient, charged with hope and dread, bears a further burden: not only disease but *surgery* causes suffering. To repeat what one surgeon told me: "Surgery is the only field that makes them sicker before you make them better."[5] What the surgeon does to the patient, *for* the patient, causes pain and suffering. This suffering—from the operation and its aftermath—does not *necessarily* lead to cure. One becomes sicker whether or not the operation makes one better.

This, too, is bitter knowledge—acquired in a terrible school. In a random universe, where God is perceived as absent or dead, the basic human questions posed in response to pain and suffering—why? why me?—echo without answer. Rather than confronting the tyranny of chance, the meaninglessness of fate, it is perhaps less agonizing for patients and their families to conclude, with the Azande, that "death always has a cause, and no man dies without a reason."

Distrust and blame then enter the picture. Both, however, have their costs.

Distrust interferes with care—and with caring. It is difficult for doctors to care for distrustful patients, and still more

difficult to care *about* them. Yet such caring may foster healing and cure. When I asked surgeons whether caring about a
patient improves surgical results, 62 percent said that it did.
Let us recall some of the reasons they advanced (Chapter 1,
pages 26–28). Several said that caring *about* patients made
them more cooperative when their surgeons cared *for* them:
caring encourages patients to participate in the painful activities that facilitate postoperative recovery. "The patient is active
after surgery, is coughing after surgery, is walking after surgery," said a European surgeon, adding, "Ah, you see, patients
hate to feel that they are considered [merely] as bodies." "The
patient feels more encouraged, rather than feeling like a slab
of meat," declared another. A third ventured that the positive
effects of physicians' caring might have to do with endorphins
(chemicals released in the brain, which decrease discomfort
and increase well-being). "I don't see how you can get people
well otherwise; it's accidental without that!" affirmed one surgeon, who described how he taught students to sit on patients'
beds and touch them caringly.

Caring cannot occur in a vacuum; it unfolds during the
interaction between patient and surgeon. Caring is not something a surgeon does *to* a patient; it takes place *between* two
unique human beings. Caring relationships are reciprocal and
mutually reinforcing: trust elicits caring, which elicits trust.
"Sometimes they'll give you tentative trust," explained the
Compassionate Young Surgeon (Chapter 5), "which you can
then earn through your behavior, and it will grow."[6]

Active distrust is chilling. It is difficult to sit on the bed of a
hostile, distrustful patient and touch that person caringly. It's
probably impossible to attempt such behavior more than once.
A patient who distrusts doctors is more likely to be treated
merely as a body and, therefore, to feel like a slab of meat.
Slabs of meat are unlikely candidates for miracles; miracles
work by means of human faith and trust.

Blame, too, has a price. In Chapter 8, I examined some

of the emotional and financial costs—to patients and doctors—of attempting to blame and punish doctors for patients' misfortunes.

Many critics assume that people have a *right* to wellness, that unworked miracles were wrongfully (and intentionally) withheld. Much rhetoric in the United States today implies such rights—and wrongs. This "critical" neo-Marxist approach is profoundly optimistic, indeed utopian: health, function, and fulfillment are perceived as there for the getting—for the giving—were they not withheld by a "bad-faith community."[7] Advocates, in a kind of Manichean duality, divide the world into the forces of good faith and bad. If health is the "natural" state of humankind, the task of the radical reformer is to attack the unholy medical and political alliance that robs unfortunates of their "natural" entitlements.

A less extreme response to doctors' untrustworthiness and uncaringness, to their depersonalization of patients, is the effort to rationalize and depersonalize the doctor-patient relationship. Proponents insist upon a basic minimum of catalogable, explicable, legislatible characteristics of the interactions between doctors and patients, to be enforced by custom, contract, and law. When the consumer movement is mapped upon the relationship between doctors and patients, doctors become "vendors" or "health-care providers" and patients, "consumers." Vendors display their wares, consumers shop with care, violations of good business practice are reported and punished. Here we have the bare-bones minimum of what is to be expected from each party to the transaction— the doctor, in particular. Included is an effort to disempower the doctor, in a bid to equalize the potentially dangerous power differential between doctor and patient.

This move toward rationalization and depersonalization of the relationship—where doctors are conceptualized as interchangeable cogs, patients as equivalent units—abandons all hope for healing and miracles. In healing, the doctor uses his or her person to reach out to the person of the patient; both are conceived of as unique—and uniquely human. Surrendering uniqueness and personhood, we relinquish the hope, faith, and healing alliance that empower miracles. Hope cannot be dashed when no hope exists. Charlatanry cannot masquerade as mystery when mystery is disenchanted. Faith cannot fail when no faith exists in a profession that is perceived as faithless.

In a rationalized, depersonalized relationship, we relinquish the possibility of the surgeon's giving of himself, of his displaying a caring and concern that can neither be bought nor legislated (as does the Compassionate Young Surgeon). We discourage the intensely *personal* devotion of the surgeon to the welfare of his patients.

While interviewing surgeons, I inquired whether I had omitted any significant questions, and one responded that I had not asked about waking up at night, explaining: "The cause of sleepless nights is not because you're too busy and not because you have lots of operations. Every once in a while you wonder if you carried out the right operation, you wonder if you did the right thing for that patient. . . . Every once in a while you say, 'What a jerk I am, I should have. . . .'" Another reported: "I always do each operation three times. I do it the night before. I do it at the operating table. And I do it the night afterwards." Others indicated similar wakefulness and worry.[8] Such watchfulness, self-monitoring, and concern about doing the right thing fits poorly into the *caveat emptor* framework of the vendor-consumer relationship.

Caring and healing do not belong to the realm of commercial contract; they are found, instead, in what theologian William May calls the "domain of *covenant*." Says May: "As opposed to a marketplace contractualist ethic, the biblical notion of covenant obliges the more powerful to accept some responsibility for the more vulnerable and powerless of the two partners. It does not permit a free rein to self-interest, subject only to the capacity of the weaker partner to protect himself or herself through knowledge, shrewdness, and purchasing power."[9] The covenantal ethic, based on an exchange of promises, "emphasizes gratitude, fidelity, even devotion and care."[10] In this responsive, reciprocal relationship, doctors repay patients' trust with care and caring. Alas, gratitude and trust can have terrible costs. Venal, incompetent, vicious doctors abuse patients' trust. The paradox is bitter: the trust that facilitates miracles can be abused by the untrustworthy, yet protecting oneself against bad faith can destroy the faith that heals.

My view of life is more tragic than that of the utopians. Unlike the critical theorists, I do not perceive health and happiness as natural rights that can be regained once the human and social obstacles to their attainment are demolished. Rather than dividing reality into a struggle between the forces of good and evil, where good will prevail once evil is vanquished, I perceive a more limited universe, where sadness, illness, and suffering are as "natural" as wellness, function, and fulfillment, where every "good" has a cost. Trust may encourage healing; the cost of trust is its potential for abuse. But distrust, too, has a cost. The temperament of surgeons may help engender miracles; its cost is arrogance and, on occasion, hubris: the unrealistic belief in one's ability to produce miracles. Draconian regulations may inhibit wrongdoers; their cost is the transformation of honest and well-meaning doctors into liars. Malpractice suits may punish wrongdoers; their cost is expensive, unnecessary tests and procedures—and angry and disillusioned doctors.

Unlike the utopians, I have no easy answers. Because I do not perceive the world as locked in a struggle between the forces of good and evil where, if only we vanquish the representatives of the bad-faith community, good will prevail, I cannot propose simple solutions to complex problems. All I can do is to try to refine some of the questions we ask, so that—in place of righteous and ultimately futile anger—we can seek some (grantedly) difficult and imperfect answers.

CODA

The Research Process

What we call the beginning is often the end
And to make an end is to make a beginning.
The end is where we start from.

> T. S. Eliot
> "Little Gidding"

BEGINNINGS

*T*HE IDEA of studying surgeons originated when the editor of a professional journal asked me to write an article reviewing Charles Bosk's book on the training of young surgeons [1] and suggested that, for the article, I interview two or three senior surgeons who had read the book. Their responses were so interesting that I ended by interviewing ten. [2] In his book, Bosk described how professional self-controls are instilled in surgical house officers by the senior surgeons who train them. I wondered how such controls functioned later in a surgeon's career, when he is no longer closely supervised by superiors who insist on a high level of moral and technical performance—punishing those who cannot follow the rules and dismissing those who will not. When the surgeons I interviewed responded to my questions about who was responsible for a surgeon's moral and technical performance, and what happened at their hospital when a colleague misbehaved, I had no way to verify their responses. One man, for example, described how his testimony against two colleagues on trial for malpractice had lost him his job and made it so difficult to find another that he was forced to accept a position in another country. Was this an accurate description? Or did this surgeon omit essential details about his own behavior and relations with colleagues? Several men claimed that, although they had heard of misbehavior "elsewhere," in *their* hospital surgeons were compelled to behave with moral and technical exactitude. Was this true? Did bad things happen only at what they called "Elsewhere Hospital"? There was no way to check their allegations. To learn more, I would have to do fieldwork among surgeons for an extended period of time.

If it were possible to conduct fieldwork among surgeons, I was a logical choice to do so. I was a contemporary of the surgeons I proposed to study, had at that time been married to a doctor for twenty-four years, and knew something about a doctor's life. My husband was at the same stage in his career as the senior surgeons I proposed to study. Even the fact that I was a woman, attempting to observe a largely masculine field, could be helpful: surgeons might discount a woman and be less annoyed by her following them around asking "dumb" questions than they would be by a man.

My experience as a doctor's wife led me to believe that professional self-controls did exist—at least among some doctors. I doubted, however, that the situation as described by eight of the ten surgeons interviewed was entirely as described: that bad behavior only took place "elsewhere." I noticed that my husband would change the subject when misbehavior among his colleagues at his hospital was discussed. I suspected it made him feel so terrible that he preferred not to think about misbehavior among colleagues, denying knowledge of what occurred: "After all, how can I know what they do with their patients?"

ACCESS REFUSED

That I was married to a doctor, and receptive to their viewpoint, did not assure a welcome from the surgeons I proposed to study. I negotiated for the better part of a year with a representative of the department of surgery at the hospital where my husband was an attending physician before the chief of surgery definitively refused to allow me to study his department. At the same time, after spending six months obtaining an interview with a representative of the American College of Surgeons, I flew to Chicago to request advice and possible sponsorship from this prestigious group. After a courtly surgeon, in his sixties, indulged in an hour of small talk, I broke in and asked if he thought my study worth doing. Silence. "Your husband is a doctor?" he finally inquired. When I assented, he said: "Have you ever thought of . . . I mean, with your background, you'd be such an asset . . . Has it ever occurred to you to become active in the ladies' auxiliary of your husband's hospital?" This was the only advice I received.

After more than a year of letters, introductory interviews, and phone calls, I had still not managed to find a group of surgeons that would agree to be studied. One chief assented, but his senior surgeons refused; the seconds in command at two departments of surgery were unable to convince their chiefs to let me in; several chiefs did not respond to my letters or phone calls. A medical sociologist suggested I forget about observing surgeons and start interviewing as many as I could find. This seemed more feasible than fieldwork, but I was unsure how much more I could learn by interviewing twenty, forty, or even a hundred surgeons than from the ten interviews already carried out. I did not want to confine my research solely to interviews; the surgeons refused to be observed; the project appeared doomed.

Let me note that my subject, self-regulation; my study population, surgeons; and the time I proposed to conduct research, the early 1980s, all worked against me. Malpractice suits, awards, and insurance costs were escalating, regulations limiting surgeons' fees and autonomy were being promulgated, and "hate doctor" and "hate surgeon" tracts being circulated. Surgeons felt beleaguered. "They're all scared. They think the only thing that can happen is bad, and if you don't come, nothing can happen," explained one man, when I was turned down by a hospital where he was an attending surgeon. When Pearl Katz studied surgeons, in the late 1970s,[3] she worked in a single hospital, at the surgeons' request, to help them solve departmental problems; and she worked in Canada, a country with significantly fewer malpractice suits than the United States. Millman carried out her research (as far as I can tell) in the early 1970s; her book and others like it may have been among the factors that made my project less feasible. I asked for a lot. I wanted free access to a hospital, to be allowed to go where I wanted, observe whom I wanted, when I wanted—including operations. Several medical anthropologists told me my project did not have a chance; even if the surgeons let me in, warned one, the hospital's research review committee would keep me out. Although theoretically, such committees rule on the ethical adequacy of research, he told me, their true function is to protect the hospital, and no committee is going to want a nosy anthropologist wandering around; the hospital has too much to lose.

ENTRÉE

At almost the last moment, when a reviewer for a grant request demanded proof that I had access to surgeons, a friend of my husband's said I could study surgeons at the suburban university-affiliated community hospital where he was chief, wrote a letter to that effect, and the study was funded by the National Endowment for the Humanities.[4]

Gaining physical access was the first step. Gaining social access was as difficult, frustrating, and time-consuming as getting in. Although the first chief of surgery was tremendously helpful and supportive—running interference with the institutional review committee that had to pass on my study, obtaining a house officer's white coat to help me blend in, and allowing me to spend weeks following him around the hospital—it was months before any of the senior surgeons I wanted to study took public notice of my presence or said a word to me.

I had planned to spend ten months in the first hospital; instead, I spent eighteen. It took all this time to gain acceptance by surgeons, house officers and nurses, to begin to understand the esoteric language of surgery, filled with technical terms and abbreviations, and to learn the procedures sufficiently to be able to observe an operation while "keeping sterility" and not interfering with what was going on. I knew research was going well when four separate people gave me a blow-by-blow description of a scene I had missed, during which a temperamental surgeon had made the head operating-room nurse cry. I was told that afterwards, she remarked to another nurse, "Joan Cassell will get a whole chapter in her book from this!" (The doctors and nurses told me I was going to write a book; at the time, I was unsure what the research would produce.)

SAMPLE AND METHODS

I subsequently obtained entrée to three additional hospitals where I studied general surgeons. Thus, I studied surgeons at two community hospitals[5] and two university hospitals. In addition, I observed surgeons at ten more hospitals, two health maintenance organizations, and a union clinic.[6] I focused on general surgeons, while also observing members of other surgical specialities; I concentrated on senior surgeons, but spent time with house officers as well. I conducted formal, tape-recorded, open-ended interviews with thirty-seven surgeons: thirty senior general surgeons; one general-surgery fellow; three chiefs of surgery; and three chief residents. Because of the scarcity of senior female general surgeons, I interviewed the seven I encountered. (Every surgeon was observed at work before being interviewed. This practice allowed me to compare what the surgeons said they did on specific occasions—such as a patient insisting upon an operation they felt was unjustified—with what I observed them doing.)

Although I was given free run of the four hospitals I studied intensively, the surgeons controlled what I saw, what I heard, and what was explained to me. In order to observe anything ticklish or controversial, I had to catch little clues, look disinterested, and refrain from asking questions. Today, when I reread my field notes, I perceive how much I missed; and how much the surgeons took it for granted I would miss (when they did talk relatively freely in front of me). What they did not count on was my persistence—that I would keep on month after month, in hospital after hospital, until finally, in retrospect, some of the events in my field notes, which I recorded but did not understand, now make sense.

I found that taking field notes made surgeons, house officers, and nurses nervous and self-conscious. Therefore, I retired the field notebook used in previous projects and substituted three-by-five-inch cards[7] stashed in the pocket of my white coat or operating-room scrub suit. I took as few notes as possible, occasionally scribbling a few words to jog my memory for each night's session at the word processor, when I poured out everything I could remember about the day's occurrences.

In the first two hospitals, I observed specific settings and activities on a regular basis, then spent a day following every senior general surgeon and chief resident who allowed me to do so through his daily activities. In the second two hospitals, where I spent less time, I spent a day following every senior surgeon.[8] (I followed each surgeon wherever he or she permitted: to examining rooms during their office hours, to clinics, health maintenance organizations, additional hospitals. I was allowed to observe the surgeon operate in some hospitals; in others, I could merely follow as the surgeon made rounds.)

During thirty-three months of research, I observed more than two hundred operations. During two operations, at two different hospitals, a senior surgeon allowed me to "scrub" and hold retractors along with medical students and interns. It was terrifying and exciting. "If you let 'em cut, they all want to become surgeons," said one resident, describing how she became interested in surgery as a medical student. "The minute I got a scalpel in my hand, that was it!" she said. I never got that scalpel in my hand.

NOTES

PREFACE: SOME WORDS FOR SOCIAL SCIENTISTS

1. "Ethnography," as Michael Agar (1980:1) points out, is an ambiguous term representing both a *process*, a method of research, and a *product*, the written results of that method.

Sometimes called "fieldwork," "participant observation," or "qualitative research," ethnography is, perhaps, the basic anthropological research method. Traditionally, the anthropological field-worker lived with a remote exotic group for six months to several years, in order to penetrate their world of meanings and values. Brownislaw Malinowski's description of his entry into "the field" is classic:

> Imagine yourself suddenly set down surrounded by all your gear, alone on a tropical beach close to a native village, while the launch or dinghy which has brought you sails away out of sight. . . . Imagine yourself then, making your first entry into the village, alone or in company with your white cicerone. Some natives flock around you, especially if they smell tobacco. Others, the more dignified and elderly, remain seated where they are. (Malinowski 1961:4)

Today, anthropologists, sociologists, social psychologists, and educational researchers use ethnographic methods to study everything and everyone, from addicts (Agar 1980) to rodeos (Lawrence 1982) to desegregated schools (J. Cassell 1978) to men and women in large corporations (Kanter 1977). The field-worker may or may not live with those she studies, she may or may not supplement her observations and questions with more quantitative (numerical) techniques, but central to the method is the researcher's spending long periods of unstructured time with those studied. In fieldwork, the observer is her own measuring instrument; it is the researcher's reactions to the researched that provide data. Rather than seeking to *measure* or *predict*, the primary aim of ethnography is to *understand*. It is open-ended: the researcher goes into "the field" to examine the situation rather than clearly defining and delimiting all the relevant "variables" ahead of time. The method is frequently more time-consuming than a purely quantitative study, since the researcher cannot specify in advance the exact nature of the phenomena that will be examined, analyzed, and compared. The investigator does not enter the field with planned, and possibly arbitrary, measures and criteria; instead, the research is guided by the unfolding events in the field. As a result, fieldwork is extremely flexible. It can discover the unexpected and adapt to unforeseen and rapidly changing circumstances. It is prodigal of time and of intellectual and psychic energy, however, since the research route has not been precisely mapped in advance.

As product, an ethnography expresses, in writing, the findings of the field-worker. Ethnographic research, then, produces an ethnography, a book or scholarly monograph describing the "culture" of a specific group.

2. For examples, see Myerhoff and Ruby 1982; Clifford and Marcus 1986; Clifford 1988; Van Maanen 1988; and Rosaldo 1989.

3. See Spencer 1989:160. Rosaldo (1989:40) and Pratt (1980:33) also address this issue, as does Stoller (1989), who describes most contemporary anthropological writing as "turgid" and "sludgy."

4. Freidson 1970:179. For an insightful discussion of Freidson's approach, see Paget 1988:15–17.

5. Paget 1988:16.

6. Millman 1976.

7. Thus, when Millman (1976:72, 109) describes the way house officers and senior physicians "think about," "hold in contempt," or joke about certain patients, such as alcoholics and obese persons, disdaining them as "nondeserving" or "garbage", she neglects to note that

such patients classically do not follow directions, and that consequently, their diseases remain impervious to the doctors' efforts. The ethnographer's indignation and unquestioning identification with the "patient as victim" conceals the complexities of interaction and frustration between doctors and patients who are believed to be unwilling or unable to cooperate in their own medical care. Ordering doctors to take proper care of overweight or alcoholic patients, or even instituting sanctions for not doing so, will have little effect, unless the vexing problem of how doctors can go about caring for difficult and demanding patients who cannot or will not care for themselves is confronted. The hot glow of anger makes the ethnographer, and possibly the reader, feel wonderfully virtuous; but it conceals, rather than illuminates, the full scope of the problem, and hence, possible solutions to it.

8. Paul Stoller (1989:28–29) presents various comments by publishers and referees on his books and articles. Let me first note that Stoller is intelligent, learned, and writes superbly; he's a pleasure to read. His imagination, clarity, and descriptive power are perceived as flaws by critics, who write disparagingly: "contains some interesting data . . . but the theoretical argument was insufficiently well-developed"; "failure to meet the canons of academic evidence"; "some interesting description . . . [but] at this point it is a half-baked manuscript"; "weakness of theoretical grounding."

The reader who finds my tone defensive should be advised that I am responding to similar reactions to my own work.

9. Strathern 1987:269.

10. Strathern 1987:269.

11. Spencer 1989:159.

12. Rosaldo 1989:127–143.

13. The good-little-girl graduate students are, after all, following the advice of their Germanic professors.

14. See, for example, Rosaldo 1989.

15. The term is Geertz's (1988:49), who describes E. E. Evans-Pritchard's writings as "African transparencies." A minor ethnographic cottage industry has burgeoned, writing *about* Evans-Pritchard's writing style (for example, Geertz 1988; Clifford 1988; Rosaldo 1989; Van Maanen 1988; and Spencer 1989), which has been variously characterized as "transparent," "realist," "classic," and "naturalist." I suspect Evans-Pritchard is so frequently chosen as exemplar of a particular kind of writing, and by extension a particular kind of research, because of a kind of concealed masculine nostalgia—the critics are all men—for a pre-feminist, pre-anti-colonialist world where brave and warlike ethnographers could keep a stiff upper lip and assume the "white man's burden" without question or qualm.

16. Consider Margaret Mead. Now that she's safely dead, beatification is under way in preparation for eventual canonization. As her student, however, I observed younger male colleagues savage Mead behind her back. She had committed the ultimate sins: simplicity, understandability, achieving popular recognition. Freud's description of the killing and ritual consumption of the tribal father pales beside these young Turks' fearful gusto as they attempted to dismember and devour the mother.

17. See, for example, Riesman 1977; Rabinow 1977; Myerhoff 1978; Favret-Saada 1980; Friedrich 1986.

18. The first time one encounters the ethnographer in a book based upon her fieldwork can be startling, even embarrassing. It seems so exhibitionistic, so, well, *naked,* to present the anthropologist as an actor in the ethnographic drama. In 1976, the late Victor Turner suggested I rewrite my dissertation on the contemporary American women's movement to alter the passive locutions and place myself in the stream of events. It would have been a better book (J. Cassell 1989) if I had followed his advice.

19. Sigmund Freud (1965:318, 342–43) discusses "overdetermina-

tion," where an activity is determined by a number of different psychic elements, each of which by itself could have been responsible for the activity.

20. Rosaldo 1989:182; Walzer 1987.

21. Millman 1975:619.

INTRODUCTION: THE SURGICAL "MIRACLE"

1. Goffman 1967:149–60.

2. Goffman (1967:159) defines consequentiality as "the capacity of a payoff to flow beyond the bounds of the occasion in which it is delivered and to influence objectively the later life of the bettor."

3. Bosk 1979:122–27.

4. Lakoff and Johnson 1980:5.

5. Selzer 1976:15.

CHAPTER 1: THE ART, CRAFT, AND SCIENCE OF MIRACLES

1. An exception to this is the best-selling book *Love, Medicine and Miracles* by surgeon Bernie Siegel (1986). Siegel, however, is referring to " 'miraculous' *healings*" (Siegel 1986:21), not surgical *cures*. Patients, naturally, will accept any kind of miracles they can get, be they based upon healing or curing (Siegel discounts neither option). Surgeons, however, tend to be wary of Siegel's inspirational, somewhat mystical combination of modern surgery and faith healing.

2. These come from the surgeon's junior partner, a chief resident, a colleague, and a young surgeon just beginning private practice. All but the first are direct quotes from tape-recorded interviews, in response to the query: "Is there any surgeon at this hospital, or whom

you've known in your training or career, who typifies your ideal surgeon? What does (did) he do that you admire?" Several subsequent descriptions of admired behavior are responses to the same interview question.

3. See Gordon's (1988a:268) contrast between "practical" and "theoretical" knowledge. Her definition of practical knowledge includes my next category of clinical judgment, or expertise, which comprises the *art* as opposed to the *science* of medicine.

4. Senior surgeons question house officers about how many patients with a particular disease or injury suffer from a particular complication and how successful various operative procedures, drugs, and other treatments are in preventing or relieving various diseases, injuries, and complications (see Atkinson 1988). Responses include the name of the senior author of journal articles on the subject, the source of the citations, and the statistical outcomes of the experimental treatments.

5. Konner (1987:103) quotes a surgical saying: "When in doubt, whip it out."

6. Wound dehiscence, where the patient's incision splits open some time after the operation, is rare and dreaded.

7. E. J. Cassell 1977.

8. Bosk 1979:92.

9. The concentration exhibited by star athletes and great musicians may be similar in some respects to that of surgeons. Defeated tennis players talk of "losing their concentration," and a famous flutist, discussing teaching, said: "The biggest problem is concentration. It's very easy to hear when someone gets a phrase going and then relaxes. I tell them they can't do it that way" (*New York Times* 1988b). The performer's physical, psychic, and mental powers must be focused exclusively on the task at hand.

10. Once, during an operation, I joined two medical students in holding retractors (instruments that hold the incision open, so that the surgeon(s) can operate) for more than eight hours. I was sufficiently excited (and terrified) so that I, too, felt no hunger, thirst, or bladder pressure. Observing operations, on the other hand, I frequently left the room for coffee, water, a toilet break—as do operating-room nurses, who are replaced for coffee breaks, meals, and, at the end of their shifts. Surgeons, needless to say, do not have shifts and some have told me of operating for as long as thirteen hours without a break.

11. Edith Turner, personal communication.

12. *New York Times* 1987.

13. I have just received a fellowship from the National Endowment for the Humanities to conduct a pilot study of women surgeons. I will be studying women above the rank of house officer in every surgical subspecialty except for ophthalmology and ob-gyn.

14. I have chosen to follow the tradition in anthropology that treats field notes as original sources. Therefore, all my field notes appear as I originally wrote them with additions in brackets and deletions indicated by ellipses.

15. Thus, in the breast biopsy described on pages 19–20, Dr. Verdi took pains to conceal a scar that would be visible in bathing suits and décolleté gowns. Concealing scars and impressing patients is all very well when the procedure is simple, such as a biopsy, and the scar might be visible when the patient were clothed. However, to concentrate on such matters during a more serious operation, such as a mastectomy, would demonstrate lack of judgment and (if the surgeon were rough on tissue) lack of technical facility as well.

16. A test that shows whether the patient's body salts are balanced; if not, the composition of the fluids administered intravenously (through a tube attached to a needle in the patient's vein) can be adjusted to balance them.

17. For example, see Fabrega 1975; E. J. Cassell 1976; Eisenberg 1977; Kleinman 1978, 1980; Eisenberg and Kleinman 1981.

18. Gaines and Hahn 1985:4.

19. Helman 1985:293.

20. For a similar story, see E. J. Cassell 1976:13–14.

21. E. J. Cassell 1976.

CHAPTER 2: THE TEMPERAMENT OF SURGEONS

1. Bateson 1951:119.

2. Wolfe 1979.

3. J. Cassell 1981.

4. See E. J. Cassell 1977.

5. Selzer 1982: 40–41.

6. The temperamental differences between members of various specialties are legend among doctors. It was a surgeon who told me the following joke:

> An internist, a general practitioner, and a surgeon are hunting ducks. A duck appears and the GP says, "It looks like a duck and it flies like a duck and I'm going to call it a duck." He shoots and misses. When the second bird appears, the internist says, "It looks like a duck and flies like a duck, but we'll have to rule out the stork and the golden eagle and the whooping crane." Before he can fire, the duck flies away. When a third bird appears, the surgeon lifts his gun and fires, and the bird drops at his feet: "Well, what do you know," he says, "it's a duck!"

7. The surgeon subsequently told me that in this particular operation, an abdominal aortic aneurysectomy, the clamp has to come out fast: the longer it's left on, the more dangerous it is to the patient.

8. The term "operating theatre" is still used in Great Britain. In the American hospitals I studied, the operating room was referred to as the "OR"—but I was assured that the old term, "operating theatre," is still known. On the front cover of Bosk's book on the training of surgeons (see Bosk 1979) is a reproduction of a painting of an old-time operating theatre, by Thomas Eakens; the setting resembles a Greek ampitheatre, with the spectators in a raked bank above the stage where the operation is taking place.

9. See Broyles 1984.

10. Let me emphasize that this is the surgeon's view of the operation. Anesthesiologists do not perceive themselves as under the command of the surgeon, and in fact, anesthesiologists have the power to cancel an operation if they believe the patient cannot tolerate anesthesia at that time.

11. This is the second part of the first Hippocratic aphorism, which begins: "Life is short and the art is long, the occasion fleeting, experience fallacious, and judgement difficult."

12. Senior surgeons and house officers were more likely to gather at a table reserved for surgeons when the chief permitted them to wear scrub suits (with a covering layer) outside of the operating-room suite. In some hospitals, one had to change to street clothes before leaving the OR suite; this was sufficiently time-consuming to induce surgeons, with ten or twenty minutes to spare between procedures, to "hang out" in the OR lounge, instead. The geography of the OR suite, the rules governing surgeons, and the friendly or unfriendly atmosphere of each department of surgery, affected the data I was able to collect: where I could collect it, how, and how easily.

13. Selzer 1982:104.

14. Selzer 1982:50.

15. Van Gennep 1960; P. Katz 1981; also see Felker 1983.

16. Klass 1988.

17. Hughes 1958:97; Kluckhohn 1942:68.

18. Also, see Bosk 1979 on quasi-technical errors.

19. Eliade 1961.

20. Selzer 1982:106.

21. See Murray (1925) on the Greek mysteries, and Otto (1931) on the sacred.

22. Fox 1957.

23. Fox 1980.

24. J. Katz 1984.

25. Shapiro 1965.

26. Those who exhibit paranoid style, says Shapiro, "are not merely capable of remarkably active, intense, and searching attention; they seem essentially incapable of anything else. They are always sharp-eyed and searching, always intensely concentrating." They manifest a quality which can be described as "hyperalertness": they are ready for anything unexpected and immediately become aware of it (Shapiro 1965:59–62). These are useful characteristics for a surgeon. Again, let me emphasize that I am discussing *paranoid style* or *mode of functioning,* not "delusional paranoia" or "paranoid schizophrenia." The first is a tendency, the second a psychotic state. (I am indebted to Arthur Kleinman, who brought Shapiro's work to my attention.)

27. Shapiro is but one of the authorities who stresses the projection involved in "paranoid" feelings of persecution, where a person's own hostile or destructive impulses are ascribed to others, who are then suspected of conspiring against that person. (See Noyes and

Kolb 1959:436; American Psychiatric Association 1969:72; Fleischer 1951:295).

28. J. Katz 1984.

CHAPTER 3: THE FELLOWSHIP OF SURGEONS

1. Oxford English Dictionary, 1971 ed., s.v. "fellowship."

2. For example, for "community," see Bell, and Newby 1973; for "primary group," see Cooley 1912:23 and Acock, Dowd, and Roberts 1974; for "network," see Barnes 1954; Mitchell 1969; Harary and Norman 1965.

3. The distinction between surgery and medicine has a long history: surgeons, who descend from the medieval barber-surgeons, who pulled teeth and lanced abscesses, were disdained by the more highly educated physicians (Robinson 1984). Colonial America followed the pattern of eighteenth-century England, where physicians, as members of a learned profession, distinguished themselves from the lower orders of surgeons, who practiced a craft (Starr 1982:37).

4. Redfield 1956.

5. Surgeons tend to operate at the hospital used by the referring internist or general practitioner. The hospitalized patient can then also be visited by his or her "medical" doctor, and the two doctors can work together when necessary. Naturally, this practice also increases the pool of medical doctors who may refer patients to that surgeon.

6. Barnes 1954.

7. After an operation, surgeons dictate notes, listing every step, every difficulty, every finding; these include the specific incision(s), needle(s), and thread employed. These notes can help protect surgeons and hospitals in case of lawsuits. A constant battle is fought

between hurried surgeons, who scant this step, and hospital administrators, who threaten dire reprisals for those whose notes are not up-to-date. The hospitals I observed all had special telephones that surgeons could use for dictating postoperative notes; these were then transcribed by hospital employees.

8. All the hospitals I observed conducted weekly surgical m(ortality) and m(orbidity) conferences, where cases with negative outcomes (death or complications) were reviewed (see Bosk 1979:112–46). I found more variation in grand rounds, which traditionally "celebrate the extraordinary successes of surgeons where expectations are negative and outcomes are positive" (Bosk 1979:122). At some hospitals, grand rounds were indeed an occasion for surgeons to describe successful cases; at others, they consisted of lectures by visiting experts, following (or replacing) the weekly M and M conference.

9. Freidson and Rhea 1963.

10. J. Cassell 1981:1963.

11. To prepare ("prep") a colon (or bowel) to be operated on, the feces are evacuated through some combination of diet, drugs, and enemas. Such preparation significantly reduces the chance of postoperative infection.

12. Such literalness is self-protective. Should the surgeon with a poor reputation be denied "privileges" to operate at a particular hospital, and sue, a shrewd lawyer would be able to demonstrate that colleagues, who criticized his ability, had *not* observed him operate and were talking on the basis of "unfounded" rumors. Friends and members of the same practice group, who *had* observed the surgeon operate, would be less likely to testify against him. As for house officers—who, I suspect, are the sources of many such rumors—their careers are entirely dependent upon the recommendations of seniors, and it would be a brave, indeed reckless, house officer who would venture to testify against a senior surgeon. (Nurses, too, may originate rumors, but their credibility, in face-to-face accusations against surgeons, would not be high.)

13. A distinction exists between "university" hospitals (the primary hospital for a medical school) and "university-*affiliated*" hospitals, which have some connection with the medical school. House officers, in the training program of a university hospital, frequently "rotate" through the affiliated hospitals, spending several months working at each, as well as at the university hospital itself. Since the affiliated hospitals are in the same area, the "grapevine" extends.

14. Other social scientists have observed surgeons at work. Their primary research focus, however, was not on the surgeons, but on issues such as "role distance" (Goffman 1961:115–32) and hospital organization (Burling, Lentz, and Wilson 1956; Wilson 1954).

15. Bosk 1979.

16. Millman 1976.

17. P. Katz 1981, 1985, 1988.

18. According to the *Oxford English Dictionary* (1971 ed., s.v. "morality play"), the "morality play," or "morality," is a "species of drama (popular in the 16th c.) in which some moral or spiritual lesson was inculcated, and in which the chief characters were personifications of abstract qualities." One of the most famous of these morality plays is *Everyman* (Anonymous, late fifteenth or early sixteenth century).

19. Although this discussion applies to other specialties as well, I will concentrate here on surgical training.

20. In the United States, the "apprenticeship" begins in the final two years of medical school, where students, doing their "clinical rotations," spend several months in various departments, such as surgery, internal medicine, pediatrics, and so on. The students learn basic skills, are exposed to various career options, and help the house officers by doing "scutwork" (see Klass 1987).

21. Klass (1987:60), describing a terrified medical student perform-

ing a new procedure, notes: "In theory, someone senior to you should walk you through each procedure slowly the first time, leaving you confident and ready to do it on your own the next time." This "theory" is violated in practice, however, and frequently "See one, do one, teach one" is the frightening (to the student or house officer), painful, even dangerous (to the patient) course of events.

22. Bateson 1951:119.

23. Bosk 1979.

24. This comes from a tape-recorded interview.

25. Some years ago, a physician told me how he began psychoanalysis after having an affair with his mentor's mistress and being ferociously and explicitly denounced for his Oedipal presumptions by that mentor.

26. See May 1983:109.

27. Bosk 1979.

28. Bosk 1979:106–7.

29. Gluckman 1963.

30. J. Cassell 1981.

31. Bosk 1979:12.

32. This man is quoted more extensively in Chapter 8.

33. Bosk 1979:36–70.

34. From the anonymous fifteenth- or sixteenth-century drama, *Everyman*.

35. Lovejoy 1961.

36. Lovejoy 1961:105.

37. My thanks to Eric Cassell, who introduced me to Lovejoy's book, suggesting it might help explain self-regulation among surgeons.

38. The relationship between surgery and medicine resembles that between segmentary societies who compete, but join together against outsiders (Evans-Pritchard 1969). Within the two specialties, the resemblance continues: academic (or "full-time," salaried) surgeons and internists, who work at hospitals connected to medical schools are differentiated from practitioners; practitioners affiliated with elite hospitals are differentiated from those affiliated with uncelebrated institutions; practitioners in uncelebrated institutions who are board-certified are differentiated from those who have not passed their specialty board examinations; among practitioners who are not board-certified, graduates of American medical schools are differentiated from FMGs (foreign medical graduates). In each case, the smaller segments unite against a larger opposing segment.

CHAPTER 4: COSTING OUT MIRACLES: THE BUSINESS OF SURGERY

1. Clinic surgery, for indigent patients, also has its costs. Patients wait hours, in uncomfortable and often degrading conditions, to be seen, diagnosed, and treated. Many hospitals refuse to care for indigent patients, who are "dumped" upon public hospitals. In others, their disorders serve to train house officers, whose inexperience affects the care these patients receive.

2. Says Starr (1982:362–63):

> By the 1960s the medical profession had developed three more or less distinct sectors. First of all, there were the doctors who worked in medical schools or hospitals, including the house staff and full-time faculty, whose priorities were research and training. . . . The chief feature of their relations with patients was that they rarely had any long-term relations with them at all. Physicians in training or engaged in research do not require

their patients' good will for future business. Their professional rewards depend on the opinion of colleagues.

The second group were the private, primarily office-based practitioners who in large numbers had moved to the suburbs. Though they had lost control of some medical institutions, they still had a privileged and dominant role in community hospitals . . . they depended more on the good will of patients than did institutionally based physicians, and they also required the good will of their colleagues in private practice for referrals, staff privileges at local hospitals, and malpractice defense.

And finally, there were the doctors working in rural or inner-city areas or state institutions. Smallest in number, lowest in prestige, these were often older general practitioners or, increasingly, younger foreign medical graduates.

Each sector has a different relationship to the business of surgery.

3. The busiest surgeon performed 13.0 "hernia equivalents" weekly. (A hernia operation is used, here and elsewhere, as a comparative measure for surgical procedures in terms of operating-room time, hospitalization time, and surgical fee.) The mean weekly work load was 4.3 hernia equivalents; the median, 3.1 hernia equivalents. The surgeon who operated the least performed 0.9 weekly hernia equivalents (Hughes et al. 1972).

4. Moreover, Santora can afford the moral luxury of not wanting to get rich: surgical fees are sufficiently high for him to earn an extremely comfortable living without squeezing his patients or practice for the last dollar. I neither denigrate nor disbelieve his statements—but he was, perhaps, gilding the lily for the anthropologist.

5. Konner 1987:386. Konner notes that "the nickname long preceded the television program with a similar name."

6. These include operative notes and other relevant information about the patient's course and treatment.

7. See Konner 1987.

8. Foreign medical graduates (FMGs) are ranked lowest on the medical hierarchy of prestige. Starr (1982:360) describes how, in the late

1950s, when hospitals expanded and increased their number of house officers, American schools did not turn out enough graduates to fill the new slots:

> During the 1950s foreign medical graduates increased from 10 to 26 percent of all house staff. Initially, these doctors came primarily from Europe, but in the 1960s a major influx began from Asia, mainly Korea, India, and the Philippines. Though ostensibly in America for graduate training in hospitals, the majority chose to remain permanently. . . . In effect, the peculiar slant of American health policy (expanding hospitals, but keeping down medical enrollments) was producing a new lower tier in the medical profession drawn from the Third World.

9. I suspect I could have kept on going, found myself some "greens," and observed an operation—but I lacked the nerve and the willingness to "break sterility."

10. The Reid Hospital "grapevine" had it that, after less than two years of practice, Auerbach was earning thirty thousand dollars a month.

11. See Hughes et al. 1972:72.

12. Of course, running a candy store does not take the enormous investment of time, energy, and money that becoming a surgeon does.

13. Dr. Lan, however, was more highly respected by his colleagues than the other surgeons in his HMO—who included the hospital Buffoon. Because of his position as chief of surgery at the health plan, Lan had some leeway in scheduling patients and was able to insist on not seeing too many patients at one time. He saw thirty that day; the nurse told me that one of his colleagues had seen forty-three the previous day. The HMO surgical patients (with the exception of Lan's) were scheduled for fifteen-minute slots, thirty minutes if the surgeon performed a procedure on them in the office. This gave little time for talking. Of course, many surgeons do not converse much with patients—whether or not they work for an HMO.

14. Lan was given particular latitude in scheduling because he was chief and a highly regarded surgeon in that community.

15. Every medical school has different arrangements for the fees earned from private patients, said the chief. He indicated that, in recent years, the department of surgery (and every other academic department in a medical school) had to "earn its keep." A percentage of the money earned by the surgeons went for departmental salaries and overhead. What this meant was that, in essence, the academic doctors were competing with private practitioners for patients. I observed one hospital where this competition was ferocious: the practitioners there complained of being treated as "second-class citizens" in every area, from parking space to mortality and morbidity conferences (where the practitioners' comments were frequently ignored or subtly ridiculed) to bookings for emergency operations (where it might take several hours to several days for an emergency case to be placed on the operating-room schedule).

16. Interestingly, this young surgeon seemed to me to have a great deal of business sense: he told how he had graduated from medical school with no debts and encouraged his wife to take out a small student loan, because at 3 percent interest, he could bank the loan money and earn more than the interest they paid. Among the reasons he gave for going into academic medicine were the difficulties in starting a practice these days and his belief that most doctors will be on salary soon, so that he might as well get in "on the ground floor."

17. The department was interested in attracting a large number of patients because (1) without sufficient patients, house officers would not be given sufficient experience doing various kinds of operations; and (2) a percentage of the fees from the academic surgeons' "private" patients went to support the department.

18. A survey sponsored by the Association of American Medical Colleges indicated that approximately 80 percent of all medical school graduates owe money, and that, in 1989, the mean debt for each graduate was forty-two thousand dollars. (*New York Times*, 1990a).

I discussed finances with one surgeon, who had finished her residency the previous year. She was employed by a practitioner with the understanding that if and when it was possible, she would be made a partner. Her salary was forty-five thousand dollars a year; she owed twenty-two thousand dollars. Her husband, a pediatrician, had finished his training a year and a half before (at the same highly regarded program where she was trained). His salary from a pediatric practice group was fifty thousand dollars; he owed twenty-four thousand dollars. She said she knew they would never be rich but thought they were lucky compared with some of their friends, who owed more than fifty thousand dollars each; none of them is going to see that kind of money, she said, unless they go into some sort of business or are able to invest money. Discussing business ventures proposed by her hospital, she said, plaintively, "All I want to do is practice surgery!"

Another young surgeon, whose peers told me he was "brilliant," had gone into private practice a year and a half before we talked about the expenses of "going out on your own." His salary, from a part-time job, was thirty thousand dollars a year; his malpractice insurance cost eighteen thousand dollars and would probably go up to more than thirty thousand the following year. "I try to cut costs as much as possible," he said. He rents a furnished office for one day a week, at two hundred dollars a month; employs a secretary for three hours a week, at one hundred dollars a month (he does most of the billing himself and answers the phone when the secretary is absent); his "beeper" and answering service cost a hundred dollars a month; his telephone bill is about seventy or eighty dollars a month; then, he must pay for supplies and stationery. He and I estimated that he spent approximately six thousand dollars a year on office expenses, plus eighteen thousand dollars for malpractice insurance. This gave him six thousand dollars a year, plus whatever he earned from operations, for him, his wife (who spoke little English and did not work), and his two children to live on.

19. The number of surgeons in the United States grew from about 58,000 in 1970 to approximately 106,000 in 1985. Although the number of operations grew proportionately in the 1970s, the count has leveled off and perhaps even decreased slightly. Consequently, from 1982 to 1985, the number of operations performed by the average general surgeon fell 25 percent. (See Rutkow 1989 and American College of Surgeons 1989.) More than half of the surgeons surveyed by the American College of Physicians in 1987 felt there were too many surgeons in their community (*New York Times* 1989).

20. With few exceptions, the most financially successful surgeons I observed were, indeed, older, American-born, white men; these were the men who made the "megabucks."

21. These changes are comparatively recent, however. Surgeons, as a group, are still extraordinarily well reimbursed for their efforts: in 1988 the average annual income for a surgeon, after expenses and before taxes, was $207,500 (*New York Times* 1990a).

22. See Starr 1982.

CHAPTER 5: A DAY WITH A COMPASSIONATE YOUNG SURGEON

1. I knew a surgeon who took a partner after twenty years of solo practice. The new partner seemed competent and dedicated, but after some years, several female patients told the surgeon that his partner had made sexual advances to them. When this was verified, the surgeon, at great financial and emotional cost, severed the partnership agreement. To his surprise, a number of his long-term female patients left him for the partner. We might call this a "worst-case scenario." Nevertheless, it did occur.

CHAPTER 6: LET'S GO FOR IT!

1. Describing the doctor-patient relationship in Italy, Gordon and Allamani (1989) observe: "The physician makes the decisions; obedience rather than decision form the basis of patient participation. . . . The patient is not a partner . . . and while faith is essential, it is mediated through faith in authority (the physician), not one's own understanding."

CHAPTER 7: DEADLY SURGICAL SINS

1. The relationship between misbehavior and malpractice suits is complex, ambiguous, and at times, almost random. A recent study

by Harvard University of thirty-one thousand patients hospitalized in 1984 in New York State showed that only one out of ten (9.6 percent) of the 1 percent of patients who suffered injury as a result of medical negligence filed lawsuits. Moreover, the majority of these were for cases which the researchers concluded there had been no adverse event or no negligence (Hiatt 1990).

2. See Millman 1976 and P. Katz 1981, 1985, 1988.

3. The more questions I asked at such times, the more protective surgeons, house officers and nurses became, and the less I was able to learn.

4. Disguising people and happenings is an anthropological tradition. Nevertheless, I could have informed someone when I observed possible misbehavior or malpractice. I did not. Naturally, this decision had moral ramifications. I felt that it was more important to identify, understand, and explain surgeons' misbehavior than to inform on individual wrongdoers. I am comfortable with this decision, although another observer might have found a different posture more suitable. (Had I cast myself as a watchdog, I would have found it difficult to identify just what went on and what were its implications. I had too little technical knowledge to understand the significance of various actions without explanation from more informed observers.)

5. Millman 1976.

6. P. Katz 1981, 1985, 1988.

7. See Aristotle 1931:II.6–II.9. For a summary of Aristotle's views, see MacIntyre 1966:57–83. For a deeper analysis and provocative discussion of these and related issues, see MacIntyre 1981:chapters 12–16.

8. Jonas 1984:36.

9. In this case, the good, or goods, would be avoiding a procedure—a colostomy—that the patient would have found dirty and profoundly

humiliating, and also avoiding the genuine hazards of two additional anesthesias.

10. E. J. Cassell (1986) builds on Jonas's discussion to argue against the go-for-broke mentality of repeated attempts to resuscitate intensive-care-unit patients who have no probability of recovering sufficiently to be discharged from the hospital.

11. See Aristotle 1931:II.6–2.9; MacIntyre 1966:57–83; and MacIntyre 1981:chapters 12–16.

12. I suspect the case would have been handled differently at a university hospital.

13. This is what senior surgeons were driving at when they told me they wished a particular house officer, whose judgment and skills they rated highly, were more "aggressive" (see page 41).

14. Trauma surgery, treating injuries from mechanical or physical agents—such as guns, knives, bayonets, and automobiles—is usually performed on an emergency basis. It is gory, thrilling, and technically demanding, giving surgeons the opportunity to perform spectacular "saves." Although general surgeons operate on trauma victims, trauma is gradually becoming a separate surgical subspecialty.

15. When I inquired, in a tape-recorded interview, what he did when a patient insisted on an operation that he believed to be unnecessary, Villar responded: "I tell them I think it's unnecessary. I explain the risk-benefit ratio. I say that if it were me or my family member I wouldn't recommend it. If they are insistent, I tell them to discuss it with their medical doctor. If I can't convince them, I tell them to go to someone else." He spoke with great conviction. Unfortunately, of thirty-seven surgeons I interviewed, thirty-six said the same thing with equal conviction—including some who I *knew* performed operations their colleagues believed were unnecessary (or, as surgeons say, "not indicated"). Was Villar—and the others whose colleagues considered them "knife-happy"—lying? Or did they have uncommonly lenient standards for what was "indicated"? All I can assert with con-

fidence is that some surgeons, like Villar, performed some operations that more scrupulous colleagues avoided; others performed many such. None could be considered Exemplary Surgeons; those who performed many were surely Sleazy.

16. See Kleinman 1988:194.

17. In attempting to understand why this particular variety of misbehavior is so profoundly disturbing—to surgeons, critics, and patients alike—I found medieval theological conceptions of the "seven deadly sins" helpful (see Bloomfield 1952). I am grateful to William F. May, Cary M. Maguire Professor of Ethics, Southern Methodist University, for his help with these issues.

18. J. Cassell 1981:164.

19. In my observation, it is the health-plan administrators, rather than surgeons, who dictate purchases and set up admitting and screening procedures that employ low-level personnel to decide whether or not patients' symptoms merit testing and the time and attention of a senior surgeon. This "gatekeeper" role may be filled by secretaries or receptionists, who respond to patients' telephone calls; emergency-room house officers, who are required to see and screen health-plan patients before they can be scheduled for expensive diagnostic tests and surgical attention; or nurses, who evaluate the gravity of the patient's condition before allowing that patient to be seen by a surgeon.

20. E. J. Cassell 1986:202–6.

21. The girl had been brought to the hospital by a counselor from a group home; Whiting was operating on her because he was "on call" that day. I suspect she was what is known as a "service case"— uninsured or covered by Medicaid. It is conceivable that the young surgeon, who had recently gone into private practice, would have behaved differently to a "private" patient—which would make his lack of concern even more culpable.

22. I am indebted to William F. May for this insight.

23. The American Board of Surgery, formed in 1936, examines and certifies general surgeons. Assuring minimum quality control, board certification incidently limits the number of surgeons, distinguishing between what surgeons sometimes call "boarded" surgeons, those who were unable to pass their boards, and general practitioners, who also perform surgery (Stevens 1971:238). (See Stevens for a discussion of the history and significance of specialty boards.)

24. Too frequent is house officers'—and on occasion, senior surgeons'—relish for "fascinomas," which are rare, difficult, and complex cases that test the surgeons' mettle.

25. See Paget 1982.

26. I observed one surgeon, trained at a poorly regarded overseas medical school, who, unable to pass his surgical boards, was kept on at his hospital under a "grandfather" clause (designed to protect older doctors who had practiced surgery before the days of specialization and examinations). This man, who made a modest living performing minor procedures on patients who spoke his native language, was extraordinarily, obsessively painstaking, going over every detail two or three times, and asking for help from the chief of surgery whenever he was unsure of a detail, drug, or procedure. Although I heard jokes about him, from colleagues and house officers, they seemed relatively mild—compared to the anger and disgust provoked by surgeons who did not recognize their own deficiencies.

27. Bosk 1979:36–67.

28. Bosk 1979:37–51.

29. Bosk 1979.

30. Providing such a recommendation is not as easy as it may appear. Legal decisions permit house officers to view their recommendations, and a dissatisfied resident may well decide to sue the chief of

surgery. Such a lawsuit is messy, expensive, and exceedingly time-consuming—devouring the time of the hard-pressed chief, while the discharged house officer has both time and motivation to reverse the derogatory letter or recommendation. I have observed chiefs attempting to "write between the lines"—to intimate that a resident was no good in subtle terms that would be picked up by the recipient without being litigable. I have also heard stories of house officers with rather poor recommendations who were snatched up by other training programs.

31. Millman 1976:91.

32. See Bosk 1979:51.

33. In similar fashion, I have observed a host of expensive procedures performed on patients suffering from kidney failure—all of which were reimbursed by the government—many of which I believe would never have been performed if they had not been so reimbursed.

34. I have observed training programs where trustworthiness and caring were consciously imparted, others where they were taught by example, and still others where these qualities were apparently ignored.

35. *New York Times* 1988a.

36. Although the requirements of medical practice laws and regulations differ from state to state, various statewide levels of review exist as well. These have formal or informal links with the self-administered system of professional discipline operated by state and county medical societies. In addition, federal laws and regulations have established various mechanisms to control the cost and quality of medical care, including the statewide PSRO (Professional Service Review Organization) system, composed of doctors who review the records of those accused of misbehavior (Grad 1978). Thus, layers of institutional mechanisms exist for detecting and punishing medical misbehavior.

CHAPTER 8: IT'S NO FUN ANYMORE

1. Horrified, I reported the bet to my husband, who "reassured" me. "That often happens," he said, "especially with normal appendixes—there's nothing to taking them out!"

2. For example, Nolen 1968.

3. In a poll taken by the Gallup Organization for the American Medical Association in 1989, nearly 40 percent of the 1,004 doctors surveyed indicated that they would probably or definitely would not go to medical school if they were in college today (*New York Times* 1990b).

4. See Nolen 1968.

5. Burnham (1982:1475) calls the period between 1910 and 1950, when doctors enjoyed public respect, the "golden age of medicine." I would extend the golden age into the 1960s for surgery.

6. For a brief overview of these concepts, see Gerth's and Mill's introduction to Weber 1946 (45–55) and Weber's essays "The Sociology of Charismatic Authority" (245–52) and "Bureaucracy" (196–244) in the same volume. Also see Weber 1947:358–73. My thanks to Murray L. Wax, who pointed out the relevance of Weber's ideas to my data.

7. Weber 1946:245.

8. Weber 1946:215.

9. See Weber 1958:221.

10. Gerth and Mills 1946:50.

11. See Starr 1982:363–88. The book contains a useful account of these developments and informed speculation about the future course of American medicine.

12. See Nolen 1968.

13. Few of the private practitioners I studied "signed up" for Medicaid, agreeing to participate in all its rules, regulations, and reimbursement procedures. Some said they preferred treating a patient for nothing to becoming involved with the cumbersome and irksome bureaucratic apparatus of Medicaid. I was unable to learn how many patients the surgeons I studied did, in fact, treat without reimbursement (although I overheard conversations suggesting that many did, indeed, operate on patients who could afford to pay little or nothing). I suspect the practitioners preferred to select which patients *they* chose to donate their services to. What this meant was that the surgeons made their own distinctions between, in Bernard Shaw's terms, the "deserving" and the "undeserving" poor, distinctions that enrage medical critics (who prefer that they, the critics, rather than the surgeons, select the objects of the surgeons' benevolence). The hospitals I observed had surgical clinics for patients who could not afford private care; these were staffed by house officers and supervised by practitioners, who took turns being "on call." A clinic patient who was operated on became the patient of the practitioner who was on call at the time that patient visited the clinic. Some surgeons were more energetic and conscientious than others in carrying out these supervisory tasks (required of all surgeons who had operating "privileges" at the hospital). I did not explore this subject in detail, but I gathered that the surgeons were reimbursed by Medicaid for these operations, if and when they were willing to endure the complicated Medicaid paperwork, bureaucratic strictures, and interminable delays.

Studying a public hospital in an urban ghetto area serving primarily impoverished patients, I learned that the financial, social, and emotional relationships between surgeons and patients differed significantly from those I had observed between private patients and their surgeons. Clinic patients—at the public hospital *and* the voluntary hospitals I studied—behaved quite differently toward their doctors, and I observed surgeons at public *and* voluntary hospitals distinguishing between "deserving" and "undeserving" poor patients. These distinctions seemed to be based less upon patients' financial status than upon their willingness and ability to cooperate with their doctors in their own care—as well as their courtesy to the doctors and nurses who cared for them. Frequently, the two attributes were linked: those patients who were abusive and inordinately demanding were likely to be the ones who refused to follow directions and to learn to care for their ailments.

14. A notable exception was the intensive care unit of the public hospital in an urban ghetto area, which was filled with relatively young patients recuperating from knife and gunshot wounds and MVAs (motor vehicle accidents).

15. Critics who call for socialized medicine seem unaware that, in the British system, many operations we take for granted are not offered to patients who are over the age of fifty-five. An "unnecessary" procedure may seem essential when it promises to improve one's own quality of life or to add years to the life of one's aged parent.

16. For a brief overview of some of these developments, see Ebert 1989.

17. In 1984, I heard a surgeon estimate to a colleague that compliance with a new set of Medicare regulations would take his nurses at least twenty minutes a day per patient. If his practice includes many older patients, the surgeon may have to hire an employee who specializes in filling out such forms and keeping up with the bureaucratic requirements as they are promulgated. This means that the surgeon must provide not only salary for an additional employee, but also office space and equipment.

18. Thus, various procedures surgeons believed helpful in certain situations, such as "nutritional support"—where patients in poor condition were given a nutritionally rich supplement intravenously to help "tune them up" before they were operated on—were not reimbursable (except under certain very limited conditions).

19. Although exceptions to the regs were allowed, if the proper procedures to obtain the exceptions were followed, these procedures were so complex, arbitrary, and time-consuming that most surgeons

found it simpler to falsify a patient's record, listing additional diseases and conditions, in order to justify the care they believed that patient needed. That most of these regulations were administered by nurses (who staffed the telephones and made the day-to-day decisions, which could be reversed only by filing an appeal to the doctors who supervised the nurses) made these regulations all the more galling to surgeons.

20. Weber 1946:249.

21. See J. Katz 1984.

22. Felker (1983:354) notes that there is no logical reason why nurses pass instruments to surgeons and interns hold retractors and tie knots in sutures, rather than the other way around, except for the logic of gender role differences.

23. A striking characteristic of the OR nurses I observed was their youth; almost every one was in her twenties or early thirties. I did not encounter the older experienced nurses described by Nolen (1968)— who ran their little "empires" with competence and authority, training generations of "green" house officers—except as supervisors. Today, the older, the more experienced, and the more competent the nurse, the more frequently she seems to be channeled from patient care into administration.

24. Redfield 1953:20–21. For a discussion of the moral and the technical order in regard to the care of the terminally ill, see E. J. Cassell 1974.

25. E. J. Cassell 1985:1.

26. See Parsons 1951 and Sidel and Sidel 1977.

27. Bosk (1979:103) discusses horror stories as "grotesque catalogs of all the things that can go wrong in treating patients." Doctors' horror stories can be considered a variety of this genre.

28. The statistical incidence of such occurrences is difficult to determine and almost impossible to verify. I suspect that the number of negligent, uncaring, and incompetent surgeons is about equal to the number of cheating, exploitive, litigious patients, and that the number of proceedings that exonerate culpable surgeons is roughly equivalent to those that condemn guiltless ones.

29. To give just one poignant example, from a medical anthropologist:

> A surgeon from a small hospital near her parents' home persuaded the narrator's active, alert, and competent eighty-seven-year-old father to undergo an operation that might prolong his life for several years. Despite doubts, the father acceded, without discussing the procedure with his daughter, who lived across the continent. The operation was physically successful, but resulted in severe psychic disorientation, which not only destroyed the father's cherished image of himself as a rational, competent adult, but also devoured the meager savings he and his wife had set aside for their later years. The surgeon refused to discuss the procedure or resulting psychic disorganization with the daughter, his attitude being, "What can you expect at his age?" After the father, with his daughter's help, regained his preoperative alertness, he remarked sadly, "Jen, I fear I may have robbed myself of an easy death."

30. In contrast to stories people *narrate,* the horror stories that reach the media concern the kind of spectacular misbehavior that results in a lawsuit.

31. A government study, which examined four thousand malpractice claims, determined that over 50 percent of the cases concerned surgical error and that one-third of the physicians involved in malpractice claims were surgeons (Cooper 1978). See also Zaslow 1978.

32. I am not contending that all, or even some calculable percentage, of malpractice suits are unjustified. Naturally, surgeons were not going to tell me about lawsuits that might be, in any way, justified. Unjustified suits, however, and their threat are sufficiently frequent to contribute to surgeons' malaise and loss of pleasure in their work.

33. Grad 1980:397. The article gives a legal diagnosis of malpractice,

which is a branch of the law of negligence. For a legal discussion of malpractice suits as they pertain to surgeons, see Fiscina 1989.

34. Evans-Pritchard 1976.

35. In the words of a lawyer, "Over the years, the system has moved in the direction of compensating not only for the results of negligence, but also for a variety of bad medical outcomes in situations where negligence, though asserted, is far from clear" (Grad 1980:399).

Not only the incidence of malpractice suits, but the amount of the awards, has risen. The average incidence of malpractice claims has gone from 4.8 per 100 physicians in 1981 to 15.2 in 1986; while the mean jury award of $220,000 dollars in 1975 has become $1.76 million in 1986 (American College of Surgeons 1989).

36. Malpractice lawyers receive a percentage of the money they earn for patients who sue doctors; the higher the settlement, the more they earn. Defense lawyers, on the other hand, are employed by insurance companies; how they conduct a case does not affect their remuneration. Consequently, the motivation and performance of patients' lawyers is likely to be superior to that of the lawyers who defend doctors.

CHAPTER 9: EXPECTED MIRACLES

1. While studying surgeons, I spent little time studying patients per se, for theoretical, practical, and personal reasons. Theoretically, I concentrated upon surgeons, because their viewpoint has been presented more rarely than that of patients. Practically, as a solo researcher, I found it difficult to learn the surgeons' point of view while, at the same time, determining how patients felt about what was going on. Personally, I felt discomfort at interrupting patients and their families in the midst of tragedy, fear, and the threat of death to introduce myself as an anthropologist studying surgeons, who wanted to know how they felt about their operations. It seemed to me to be unpleasantly reminiscent of television newscasters intrusively thrusting microphones into the faces of people who have just under-

gone unimaginable adversity and loss. Instead, I observed happenings quietly, wearing my white coat and being introduced to patients in whatever way each surgeon saw fit to do so. Most introduced me as "Dr. Cassell"; some explained with amusement that I was studying *them*. When patients or family members inquired, I explained who I was and what I was doing. But when they seemed uninterested I did not thrust this knowledge on them. I felt they had enough on their minds.

I did follow one woman on the day of her operation from 9:00 A.M., when her surgeon brought me to her hospital room, through the operation, at noon, to late afternoon, when she was moved from the recovery room to return to "the floor." Her surgeon explained my research ahead of time and obtained her permission for me to observe. The patient, an Italian-born, working-class woman, introduced me to her family and inquired what I thought about Margaret Mead. It was a fascinating day. More time spent with patients would have been equally compelling, but this was *not* what I was studying. I was studying surgeons' perceptions of their work and their patients, not patients' perceptions of their surgeons. That is another project.

2. The phrase "kingdom of the sick" comes from Susan Sontag. Anthropologist and cancer patient Susan DiGiacomo (1987) quotes Sontag in saying: "Illness is the night-side of life, a more onerous citizenship. Everyone who is born holds dual citizenship, in the kingdom of the well and in the kingdom of the sick." DiGiacomo (1987, 1988) used her professional skills to analyze her experiences with doctors.

3. For example, Anselm Strauss and his collaborators (1985) divide hospital care into various kinds of "work": machine, safety, comfort, sentimental, and articulation work. This formulation allows us to separate the various tasks involved in effective patient care and realize that, although it is important that every kind of work be accomplished, not every task must be addressed by the same specialist. Neither "comfort work" (attention to patients' physical pain and discomfort caused by hospitalization and medical care) nor "sentimental work" (assuaging patients' anxiety, fear, panic, or depression) must necessarily be performed by a surgeon. What is crucial is to assure that the tasks are accomplished. Specific persons or professions might be

designated to act as interface between surgeons and patients, assuming primary responsibility for comfort and sentimental work. I have been told of some such arrangements and observed one in action—a breast-cancer clinic run by skillful and compassionate nurses and social workers, who saw their job as teaching, comforting, and caring for and about patients. Naturally, assigning such "work" away from the surgeon has its own potential cost: further bureaucratizing medical care, with the assumption that the surgeon's job is to cut, the nurses' or social workers' to care.

4. Such illnesses are (1) long-term (2) uncertain (3) require proportionately large efforts at palliation and (5) tend to consist of multiple diseases (Gerson and Strauss 1975:2–18). See Strauss et. al. 1985 and Kleinman 1988.

5. Oncology does, as well; and patients' attitudes toward oncologists are, in many ways, similar to their attitudes toward surgeons (DiGiacamo 1987).

6. See Zaner 1988:310–20 on the moral implications of the relationship between those who take care and those who must trust.

7. Scheper-Hughes 1988.

8. Cynics might contend that sleepless nights are generated by fear of malpractice suits. Such fears surely exist, although a surgeon who is too fearful cannot continue to practice surgery with the requisite daring and belief in himself. I suspect that surgeons who awaken in the middle of the night are worrying about more tangible concerns—*actual* patients or ongoing malpractice suits, rather than the possibility of suit. Someone who lacked the fortitude to bear unpleasant *possibilities* would not become a surgeon.

9. May 1980:368. Also see May 1983.

10. May 1980:367.

CODA: THE RESEARCH PROCESS

1. Bosk 1979.

2. See J. Cassell 1981.

3. P. Katz 1981, 1985, 1988.

4. Grant #RH2051484.

5. Each community hospital was affiliated with a university hospital.

6. All the senior surgeons I observed were board-certified, with the exception of two men; one exception was kept on under a "grandfather clause," and the other was still trying to pass his boards. (This does not include young surgeons, who had completed their residency but were still studying for the boards.)

7. My thanks to Charles Bosk, who advised using the three-by-five-inch cards which he employed in his study of surgical house officers.

8. This strategy was inspired by that of Pearl Katz (1981, 1985, 1988), who followed six surgeons, successively, to carry out her study.

GLOSSARY

Anastomosis. A surgical joining of two hollow organs, two parts of the same organ, or two blood vessels. In an end-to-end colon anastomosis, the joining can be performed by hand, a skilled and time-consuming procedure, or by a special stapling device designed for the purpose.

Attending. A senior surgeon (above the rank of house officer or fellow) who is authorized to admit patients to a particular hospital and operate on them there.

Chief. The head of a department, such as surgery, or of a unit in a large department, such as general surgery.

Chief Resident. A house officer in the final year of postgraduate training. The chief resident teaches and supervises the other house officers and is in turn taught and supervised by attending surgeons and the chief.

Circulating Nurse. The unscrubbed circulating nurse obtains articles from their nonsterile storage place, then opens each sealed packet containing sterile articles, holding out the packet so that the gloved scrub nurse can remove the sterile object and pass it to the surgeon. During an operation, the circulating nurse moves from the OR to the OR suite to fetch and deliver instruments, equipment, tissue samples, and so forth.

Code. An emergency attempt by a team of doctors, nurses, and technicians, to resuscitate a patient who has suffered a heart or breathing stoppage. When used as a verb, it refers to the need for such resuscitation (for example, "the patient coded").

Colostomy. The temporary or permanent formation of an artificial anus by passing one end of the severed colon through an opening in the abdominal wall, so that the patient's feces are collected in a bag outside the body.

Community Hospital. A community or voluntary hospital is a not-for-profit hospital with a professed aim of community service. Such hospitals often operate on a less-than-cost basis, supported by subsidies and charitable contributions. (The community hospitals observed for this study were all affiliated with medical schools.)

ER. Emergency room.

The floor. The wards containing surgical patients.

Full-time man. A salaried physician employed by the hospital in a teaching or administrative capacity. The chief of surgery is full-time, as are many attending surgeons in university hospitals.

Grand Rounds. A weekly conference where surgeons present and discuss interesting and instructive cases. In some hospitals, the term "grand rounds" has been extended and applied to a session following the mortality and morbidity conference, where various experts lecture on diverse aspects of the art, craft, and business of surgery.

House Officer. A medical school graduate providing service to the hospital while receiving postgraduate training in a medical or surgical specialty. A general surgeon must have five years of postgraduate training. The rank of a house officer may be formally described by the number of postgraduate years since leaving medical school: PGY1, PGY2, and so forth indicate postgraduate year 1, postgraduate year 2, and so forth.

ICU. Intensive care unit, also referred to as "the unit." An area of a hospital where critically ill patients are cared for.

Infarct. An area of dead tissue in heart, brain, or lungs caused by a plugged blood vessel.

Intern.   A house officer in the first year of postgraduate training (a PGY1). See House Officer.

M and M.   Mortality and morbidity conference. A weekly conference where surgical deaths and complications are discussed.

Munchausen's Syndrome.   A psychiatric condition that leads the sick person to induce or simulate physical illness. Such a patient may inject him- or herself with bacteria, add blood to urine or stool samples, heat a thermometer to fake a fever, and so forth.

OR.   Operating room.

Public Hospital.   A hospital staffed entirely by full-time medical personnel that predominantly serves patients who cannot afford private doctors.

Resident.   A PGY2, 3, 4, or 5 (any postgraduate year beyond the first). See House Officer.

Scrubbing.   A complex and precise procedure, involving meticulously washing one's forearms, hands, and fingernails with a special sponge and soap for two to ten minutes.

Scrub Nurse.   The nurse responsible for placing sterile instruments and supplies in the surgeon's outstretched hand as needed or requested.

Teaching Hospital.   A hospital with a postgraduate training program for house officers.

Turf.   To transfer a troublesome patient to another ward, service, or hospital.

University Hospital.   The primary hospital for a medical school. Here, full-time salaried surgeons teach house officers and medical students. Although some full-time attending surgeons operate on their own "private" patients, their academic role is paramount. In addition to teaching, many academic surgeons conduct research.

BIBLIOGRAPHY

Acock, Alan C., James J. Dowd, and William L. Roberts. 1974. *The Primary Group: Its Rediscovery in Contemporary Sociology*. Morristown, N.J.: General Learning Corporation.

Agar, Michael H. 1980. *The Professional Stranger: An Informal Introduction to Ethnography*. New York: Academic Press.

American College of Surgeons. 1989. *Socioeconomic Factbook for Surgery*. Edited by Pam Politser and Evelyn Cunico. Chicago: American College of Surgeons, Socioeconomic Affairs.

American Psychiatric Association. 1969. *A Psychiatric Glossary*. 3d ed. Washington, D.C.: American Psychiatric Association.

Aristotle. 1931. *Nicomachean Ethics*. Translated by W. D. Ross. London: Oxford University Press. Originally written fourth century B.C.

Atkinson, Paul. 1988. "Discourse, Descriptions, and Diagnoses: Reproducing Normal Medicine." In *Biomedicine Examined*, edited by Margaret Lock and D. Deborah Gordon, 179–204. Dordrecht, Netherlands: Kluwer Academic Publishers.

Barnes, J. A. 1954. "Class and Committees in a Norwegian Island Parish." *Human Relations* 7:39–58.

Bateson, Gregory. 1951. *Naven: A Survey of the Problems Suggested by a Composite Picture of the Culture of a New Guinea Tribe Drawn from Three Points of View*. Stanford, Calif.: Stanford University Press. Originally published in 1936.

Bell, Colin, and Howard Newby. 1973. *Community Studies: An Introduction to the Sociology of the Local Community*. New York: Praeger Publishers.

Bloomfield, Morton W. 1952. *The Seven Deadly Sins: An Introduction to the History of a Religious Concept, with Special Reference to Medieval English Literature*. East Lansing, Mich.: Michigan State College Press.

Bosk, Charles. 1979. *Forgive and Remember: Managing Medical Failure.* Chicago: University of Chicago Press.

————. 1985. "Social Controls and Physicians: The Oscillation of Cynicism and Idealism in Sociological Theory." In *Social Controls and the Medical Profession*, edited by Judith P. Swazey and Stephen R. Scher. Boston: Oelgeschlager, Gunn & Hain.

Broyles, William. 1984. "Why Men Love War." *Esquire*, November 1984.

Burling, Temple, Edith M. Lentz, and Robert N. Wilson. 1956. *The Give and Take in Hospitals: A Study of Human Organization in Hospitals.* New York: Putnam.

Burnham, John. 1982. "American Medicine's Golden Age: What Happened to It?" *Science* 215 (March 19):1475–78.

Cassell, Eric J. 1974. "Dying in a Technological Society." *Hastings Center Studies* 2 (2):31–36.

————. 1976. *The Healer's Art.* Philadelphia and New York: J. B. Lippincott.

————. 1977. "Error in Medicine." In *The Foundations of Ethics and Its Relationship to Science.* Vol. 1, *Knowledge Value and Belief*, edited by H. Tristram Englehardt, Jr. and Daniel Callahan, 295–309. Hastings-on-the-Hudson: The Hastings Center.

————. 1985. *Talking With Patients*, Vol. 1, *The Theory of Doctor-Patient Communication.* Cambridge, Mass.: MIT Press.

————. 1986. "The Changing Concept of the Ideal Physician." *Daedalus* 115 (Spring 1986): 185–208.

Cassell, Joan. 1978. *A Fieldwork Manual for Studying Desegregated Schools.* Washington, D.C.: National Institute of Education.

————. 1981. "Technical and Moral Error in Medicine and Fieldwork." *Human Organization* 40 (2):160–68.

————. 1989. *A Group Called Women: Sisterhood and Symbolism in the Feminist Movement.* Reprint. Prospect Heights, Ill.: Waveland Press. Originally published by David McKay (Longmans), New York, 1977.

Clifford, James. 1988. *The Predicament of Culture: Twentieth-Century Ethnography, Literature, and Art.* Cambridge, Mass.: Harvard University Press.

Clifford, James, and George E. Marcus, eds. 1986. *Writing Culture: The Poetics and Politics of Ethnography.* Berkeley: University of California Press.

Cooley, Charles H. 1912. *Social Organization.* New York: Scribner's.

Cooper, J. K., ed. 1978. *Medical Malpractice Claims.* Washington, D.C.: U.S. Department of Health, Education, and Welfare.

DiGiacomo, Susan. 1987. "Biomedicine as a Cultural System: An Anthropologist in the Kingdom of the Sick." In *Encounters with Biomedicine: Case Studies in Medical Anthropology,* edited by Hans A. Baer, 315–46. Montreaux, Switzerland: Gordon and Breach.

———. 1988. "Metaphor as Illness: Body, Mind, and the Interpretation of Disorder." Paper presented at the annual meetings of the Society for Applied Anthropology, Tampa, Florida, April 20–24, 1988.

Dostoyevski, Fyodor. [ca. 1880] *The Brothers Karamazov.* Translated by Constance Garnett. New York: Modern Library.

Drane, James F. 1988. *Becoming a Good Doctor: The Place of Virtue and Character in Medical Ethics.* Kansas City, Mo.: Sheed and Ward.

Ebert, Paul A. 1989. "Implications of Federal Legislation for Surgical Practice." In *Socioeconomics of Surgery,* edited by Ira M. Rutkow. St. Louis: C. V. Mosby.

Eisenberg, Leon. 1977. "Disease and Illness: Distinctions between Professional and Popular Ideas of Sickness." *Culture, Medicine and Psychiatry* 1:9–23.

Eisenberg, Leon, and Arthur Kleinman, eds. 1981. *The Relevance of Social Science for Medicine.* Dordrecht, Netherlands: D. Reidel.

Eliade, Mircea. 1961. *Images and Symbols: Studies in Religious Symbolism.* Translated by Philip Mairet. New York: Sheed and Ward.

Eliot, T. S. 1971. "East Coker" and "Little Gidding." In *Four Quartets.* New York: Harcourt Brace Jovanovich (Harvest Books). Originally published in 1943.

Evans-Pritchard, E. E. 1969. *The Nuer: A Description of the Modes of Livelihood and Political Institutions of a Nilotic People.* New York: Oxford University Press. Originally published in 1940.

———. 1976. *Witchcraft, Oracles and Magic among the Azande.* Abridged by Eva Gillies. Oxford, England: Oxford University Press. Originally published in 1937.

Everyman and Medieval Miracle Plays. 1956. New York: Dutton, Everyman's Library. Originally from late fifteenth or early sixteenth century.

Fabian, Johannes. 1983. *Time and the Other: How Anthropology Makes Its Object*. New York: Columbia University Press.

Fabrega, Horacio. 1975. "The Need for an Ethnomedical Science." *Science* 189:969–75.

Favret-Saada, Jeanne. 1980. *Deadly Words: Witchcraft in the Bocage*. Cambridge, England: Cambridge University Press.

Felker, Marcia Elliott. 1983. "Ideology in the Operating Room." In *The Anthropology of Medicine: From Culture to Method*, edited by Lola Romanucci-Ross, Daniel E. Moerman, and Laurence R. Tancredi, 349–65. South Hadley, Mass.: Bergin & Garvey.

Fiscina, Sal. 1989. "The Surgeon in Court." In *Socioeconomics of Surgery*, edited by Ira M. Rutkow. St. Louis: C. V. Mosby.

Fleischer, Joachim. 1951. *Mental Health and the Prevention of Neurosis*. New York: Liveright.

Fox, Renée. 1957. "Training for Uncertainty." In *The Student Physician*, edited by Robert Merton, George Reader, and Patricia Kendall, 217–41. Cambridge, Mass.: Harvard University Press.

———. 1980. "The Evolution of Medical Uncertainty." *Milbank Memorial Fund Quarterly* 1:1–49.

Freidson, Eliot. 1970. *Profession of Medicine: A Study of the Sociology of Applied Knowledge*. New York: Dodd Mead & Company, Inc.

———. 1975. *Doctoring Together*. New York: Elsevier.

Freidson, Eliot, and Buford Rhea. 1963. "Processes of Control in a Company of Equals." *Social Problems* 11:119–31.

Freud, Sigmund. 1965. *The Interpretation of Dreams*. Translated by James Strachey. New York: Avon Discus Books. Originally published in 1900.

Friedrich, Paul. 1986. *The Princes of Naranja: An Essay in Anthrohistorical Method*. Austin, Tex.: University of Texas Press.

Gaines, Atwood, and Robert A. Hahn. 1985. "Among the Physicians: Encounter, Exchange and Transformation." In *Physicians of Western Medicine: Anthropological Approaches to Theory and Practice*. Dordrecht, Netherlands: D. Reidel.

Garrison, Fielding H. 1929. *An Introduction to the History of Medicine*. Philadelphia: W. B. Saunders.

Geertz, Clifford. 1988. *Works and Lives: The Anthropologist as Author*. Stanford, Calif.: Stanford University Press.

Gerson, Elihu, and Anselm Strauss. 1975. "Time for Living." *Social Policy* 6:12–18.

Gerth, H. H., and C. Wright Mills. 1946. "Intellectual Orientations."
Introduction to *From Max Weber: Essays in Sociology*, translated
by H. H. Gerth and C. Wright Mills, 45–74. New York: Oxford
University Press. Essays originally published in 1924.

Gluckman, Max. 1963. "Gossip and Scandal." *Current Anthropology* 4
(3):307–16.

Goffman, Erving. 1961. "Role Distance." In *Encounters: Two Studies in
the Sociology of Interaction*, 85–152. Indianapolis: Bobbs-Merrill.

———. 1967. "Where the Action Is." In *Interaction Ritual: Essays on
Face to Face Behavior*. New York: Doubleday Anchor Books.

Gordon, Deborah R. 1988a. "Clinical Science and Clinical Expertise."
In *Biomedicine Examined*, edited by Margaret Lock and Deborah
Gordon, 257–95. Dordrecht, Netherlands: Kluwer Academic
Publishers.

———. 1988b. "Tenacious Assumptions in Western Medicine." In
Biomedicine Examined, edited by Margaret Lock and Deborah
Gordon, 19–56. Dordrecht, Netherlands: Kluwer Academic
Publishers.

Gordon, Deborah R., and Allaman Allamani. 1989. "Not to Tell, Not
to Know: Culture, Cancer and Communication in Italy." Paper
presented at the annual meetings of the American Anthropological Association, Washington, D.C., November 1989.

Grad, Frank P. 1978. "The Antitrust Laws and Professional Discipline
in Medicine." *Duke Law Review* 2:443–86.

———. 1980. "Medical Malpractice and Its Implications for Public Health." In *Legal Aspects of Health Policy: Issues and Trends*,
edited by Ruth Roemer and George McKray. Westport, Conn.:
Greenwood Press.

Gregory the Great. 1845. *Morals on the Book of Job*. Oxford: John Henry
Parker, and London: F. and J. Rivington.

Harary, F., and R. Z. Norman. 1965. *Graph Theory as a Mathemati-
cal Model in Social Sciences*. Ann Arbor: University of Michigan
Institute for Social Research.

Helman, Cecil G. 1985. "Disease and Pseudo-Disease: A Case History
of Pseudo-Angina." In *Physicians of Western Medicine: Anthropological Approaches to Theory and Practice*. Dordrecht, Netherlands:
D. Reidel.

Henry, Jules. 1963. *Pathways to Madness*. New York: Random House.

Hiatt, Howard. 1990. "Patients, Doctors, and Lawyers: Medical Injury, Malpractice Litigation and Patient Compensation in New York." Cambridge, Mass.: Harvard Medical Practice Study.

Hughes, Edward F. X., Victor R. Fuchs, John E. Jacoby, and Eugene M. Lewit. 1972. "Surgical Workloads in a Community Practice." *Surgery* 71 (3):315–27.

Hughes, Everett C. 1958. "Mistakes at Work." In *Men and Their Work*, 88–101. Glencoe, Ill.: Free Press.

————. 1971. "Mistakes at Work." In *The Sociological Eye: Selected Papers on Work, Self and the Study of Society*, 316–25. Chicago and New York: Aldine-Atherton.

Jonas, Hans. 1984. *The Imperative of Responsibility*. Chicago: University of Chicago Press.

Kanter, Rosabeth Moss. 1977. *Men and Women of the Corporation*. New York: Basic Books.

Katz, Jay. 1984. *The Silent World of Doctor and Patient*. New York: Free Press.

Katz, Pearl. 1981. "Ritual in the Operating Room." *Ethnology* 20 (4):335–50.

————. 1985. "How Surgeons Make Decisions." In *Physicians of Western Medicine: Anthropological Approaches to Theory and Practice*, edited by Robert A. Hahn and Atwood D. Gaines. Dordrecht, Netherlands: D. Reidel.

————. 1988. "Traditional Thought and Modern Western Surgery." *Social Science and Medicine* 26 (12):1175–81.

Klass, Perri. 1987. *A Not Entirely Benign Procedure*. New York: Signet Books.

————. 1988. "Are Women Better Doctors?" *New York Times Magazine*, April 10.

Kleinman, Arthur. 1978. "Concepts and a Model for the Comparison of Medical Systems as Cultural Systems." *Social Science and Medicine* 12:85–93.

————. 1980. *Patients and Healers in the Context of Culture*. Berkeley: University of California Press.

————. 1988. *The Illness Narratives: Suffering, Healing, and the Human Condition*. New York: Basic Books.

Kluckhohn, Clyde. 1942. "Myths and Rituals: A General Theory."
    Harvard Theological Review 35 (1):45–79.
Konner, Melvin. 1987. *Becoming a Doctor*. New York: Penguin Books.
Lakoff, George, and Mark Johnson. 1980. *Metaphors We Live By*. Chi-
    cago: University of Chicago Press.
Lawrence, Elizabeth Atwood. 1982. *Rodeo: An Anthropologist Looks at
    the Wild and the Tame*. Knoxville, Tenn.: University of Tennes-
    see Press.
Lovejoy, Arthur O. 1961. *Reflections on Human Nature*. Baltimore, Md.:
    Johns Hopkins Press.
MacIntyre, Alasdair. 1966. *A Short History of Ethics*. New York: Mac-
    millan.
———. 1981. *After Virtue*. Notre Dame, Ind.: University of Notre
    Dame Press.
Malinowski, Bronislaw. 1961. *Argonauts of the Western Pacific: An
    Account of Native Enterprise and Adventure in the Archipelagoes
    of Melanesian New Guinea*. New York: E. P. Dutton. Originally
    published in 1922.
Marcus, George, and Dick Cushman. 1982. "Ethnographies as Texts."
    Annual Review of Anthropology 11:25–69.
Marcus, George E., and Michael M. J. Fischer. 1986. *Anthropology as
    Cultural Critique: An Experimental Moment in the Human Sciences*.
    Chicago: University of Chicago Press.
Mascia-Lees, Frances, Patricia Sharpe, and Colleen Ballerino Cohen.
    1989. "The Postmodernist Turn in Anthropology: Cautions
    from a Feminist Perspective." *Signs* 15 (1):7–33.
Mathews, Joan J. 1987. "Fieldwork in a Clinical Setting: Negotiat-
    ing Entrée, the Investigator's Role and Problems of Data Col-
    lection." In *Encounters with Biomedicine: Case Studies in Medical
    Anthropology*, edited by Hans A. Baer, 295–314. Montreaux,
    Switzerland: Gordon and Breach.
May, William F. 1980. "Doing Ethics: The Bearing of Ethical Theories
    on Fieldwork." *Social Problems* 27 (3):358–70.
———. 1983. *The Physician's Covenant: Images of the Healer in Medical
    Ethics*. Philadelphia: Westminster Press.
Miller, S. M. 1952. "The Participant Observer and 'Over-Rapport.'"
    American Sociological Review 17 (1):97–99.

Millman, Marcia. 1975. Review of *The Courage to Fail: A Social View of Organ Transplants and Dialysis*, by Renée Fox and Judith Swazey. *Contemporary Sociology* 4 (6):617–19.

———. 1976. *The Unkindest Cut: Life in the Backrooms of Medicine*. New York: William Morrow.

Mitchell, J. Clyde, ed. 1969. *Social Networks in Urban Situations*. Manchester, England: University of Manchester Press.

Murray, Gilbert. 1925. *Five Stages of Greek Religion*. Oxford, England: Clarendon Press.

Myerhoff, Barbara. 1978. *Number Our Days*. New York: E. P. Dutton.

Myerhoff, Barbara, and Jay Ruby. 1982. Introduction. In *A Crack in the Mirror: Reflexive Perspectives in Anthropology*, edited by Jay Ruby, 1–35. Philadelphia: University of Pennsylvania Press.

New York Times. 1987. "Women As Surgeons: Fighting for Success." June 19.

———. 1988a. "Doctors Can Sue in Peer Reviews, Justices Declare." May 17.

———. 1988b. "Galway Uncovers Risks in Leading Charmed Life." July 16.

———. 1989. "Innovations Intensify Glut of Surgeons." November 7.

———. 1990a. "Changes in Medicine Bring Pain to Healing Profession." February 18.

———. 1990b. "Many in Medicine Are Calling Rules a Professional Malaise." February 19.

Nolen, William A. 1968. *The Making of a Surgeon*. New York: Random House.

Noyes, Arthur P., and Lawrence C. Kolb. 1959. *Modern Clinical Psychiatry*. 5th ed. Philadelphia: W. B. Saunders.

Otto, Rudolf. 1931. *The Idea of the Holy: An Inquiry into the Non-Rational Factor in Its Relation to the Rational*. 9th ed. Translated by John W. Harvey. London: Oxford University Press.

Paget, Marianne. 1982. "Your Son Is Cured Now; You May Take Him Home." *Culture, Medicine and Psychiatry* 6:237–59.

———. 1988. *The Unity of Mistakes: A Phenomenological Interpretation of Medical Work*. Philadelphia: Temple University Press.

Parsons, Talcott. 1951. *The Social System*. New York: Free Press.

Pratt, Mary Louise. 1980. "Fieldwork in Common Places." In *Writing Culture: The Poetics and Politics of Ethnography*, edited by James

Clifford and George E. Marcus. Berkeley: University of California Press.

Rabinow, Paul. 1977. *Reflections on Fieldwork in Morocco.* Berkeley and Los Angeles: University of California Press.

Redfield, Robert. 1953. *The Primitive World and Its Transformations.* Ithaca, N.Y.: Cornell University Press.

———. 1956. *The Little Community.* Chicago: University of Chicago Press.

Riesman, Paul. 1977. *Freedom in Fulani Social Life: An Introspective Ethnography.* Chicago: University of Chicago Press.

Robinson, James O. 1984. "The Barber-Surgeons of London." *Archives of Surgery* 119:1171–75.

Rosaldo, Renato. 1989. *Culture and Truth: The Remaking of Social Analysis.* Boston: Beacon Press.

Rutkow, Ira M., ed. 1989. *Socioeconomics of Surgery.* St. Louis: C. V. Mosby.

Scheper-Hughes, Nancy. 1988. "The Madness of Hunger: Sickness, Delirium, and Human Needs." *Culture, Medicine, and Psychiatry* 12 (4):429–58.

Selzer, Richard. 1976. *Mortal Lessons: Notes on the Art of Surgery.* New York: Simon and Schuster, Touchstone Books.

———. 1982. *Letters to a Young Doctor.* New York: Simon and Schuster, Touchstone Books.

Shapiro, David. 1965. *Neurotic Styles.* New York: Basic Books.

Sidel, Ruth, and Victor Sidel. 1977. *A Healthy State: An International Perspective on the Crisis in United States Medical Care.* New York: Pantheon Books.

Siegel, Bernie S. 1986. *Love, Medicine and Miracles: Lessons Learned about Self-Healing from a Surgeon's Experience with Exceptional Patients.* New York: Harper & Row.

Siegler, Mark. 1979. "Clinical Ethics and Clinical Medicine." *Archives of Internal Medicine* 139:914–15.

Spencer, Jonathan. 1989. "Anthropology as a Kind of Writing." *Man* 24 (1):145–64.

Starr, Paul. 1982. *The Social Transformation of American Medicine: The Rise of a Sovereign Profession and the Making of a Vast Industry.* New York: Basic Books.

Stevens, Rosemary. 1971. *American Medicine and the Public Interest.* New Haven: Yale University Press.

Stoller, Paul. 1989. *The Taste of Ethnographic Things: The Senses in Anthropology.* Philadelphia: University of Pennsylvania Press.

Strathern, Marilyn. 1987. "Out of Context: The Persuasive Fictions of Anthropology." *Current Anthropology* 3:251–70.

Strauss, Anselm, Shizuko Fagerhaugh, Barbara Suczek, and Carolyn Wiener. 1985. *Social Organization of Medical Work.* Chicago: University of Chicago Press.

Swazey, Judith, and Renée Fox. 1976. *The Courage to Fail: A Social View of Organ Transplants and Dialysis.* Chicago: University of Chicago Press.

Van Gennep, Arnold. 1960. *The Rites of Passage.* Translated by Monika B. Vizedom and Gabrielle L. Caffee. Chicago: University of Chicago Press. Originally published in 1909.

Van Maanen, John. 1988. *Tales of the Field: On Writing Ethnography.* Chicago: University of Chicago Press.

Walzer, Michael. 1987. *Interpretation and Social Criticism.* Cambridge, Mass.: Harvard University Press.

Weber, Max. 1946. *From Max Weber: Essays in Sociology.* Translated by H. H. Gerth and C. Wright Mills. New York: Oxford University Press. Originally published in 1924.

——. 1947. *The Theory of Social and Economic Organization.* Translated by A. M. Henderson and Talcott Parsons. New York: Oxford University Press. Originally published in 1924.

——. 1958. *The Protestant Ethic and the Spirit of Capitalism.* Translated by Talcott Parsons. New York: Scribner's. Originally published in 1904–5.

Williams, Guy. 1987. *The Age of Miracles: Medicine and Surgery in the Nineteenth Century.* Chicago: Academy Chicago Publishers.

Wilson, Robert N. 1954. "Teamwork in the Operating Room." *Human Organization* 12:9–14.

Wolfe, Tom. 1979. *The Right Stuff.* New York: Random House.

Zaner, Richard M. 1988. *Ethics and the Clinical Encounter.* Englewood Cliffs, N.J.: Prentice Hall.

Zaslow, J. 1978. "What Is Malpractice in General Surgery?" In *Legal Medicine Annual,* edited by C. H. Hecht. New York: Appleton-Century-Crofts.

INDEX

Academic surgeons, 13, 14, 16, 27, 66, 69, 78, 100–101, 131, 148, 161, 184, 192
Aggressiveness. *See* Surgical temperament
Aging, 20–21, 147, 180
American College of Surgeons, 221
Aristotle, 9, 153
Arrogance. *See* Surgical temperament
Attitudes toward doctors, changing. *See* Changing attitudes toward doctors
Auerbach, Dr. *See* Surgeons
Author as positioned subject, xxiii–xxv
Authorial voice, xix–xxi
Azande, 203, 214

Bad results, relationship of to malpractice, 154
Battle (against disease and death), 35, 38, 55, 56, 58, 185, 197
Blame, xvii, 194, 199, 203, 212–13, 214–16; price of, 215
Bosk, Charles, 16, 66, 67, 69, 70, 72, 173, 175
Breast biopsy, 19–20, 105, 169–70, 173–74
Bryna, Dr. *See* Surgeons
Buffoon. *See* Cast of characters (in morality play); Surgeons: Dr. Sutton

Carelessness. *See* Deficiencies
Caring, 21, 24, 25–28, 212–13, 215, 217; caring for vs. caring about patients, 25–28, 169, 208, 215; measuring caring behavior, 169–71; teaching caring, 26, 27, 180. *See also* Cast of characters (in morality play): Compassionate Young Surgeon; Defects, or character flaws: lack of caring
Cast of characters (in morality play), 71–72; Buffoon, 72, 74, 173–75, 180, 195; Clown, 73; Compassionate Young Surgeon, 72, 104–27; Everyman, 60, 76; Exemplary Surgeon, 32, 72, 75, 77–78, 85–87, 98–100, 198, 202; Old-Time Surgeon, 72, 85–87, 128–52; Prima Donna, 72, 73, 75, 128–52, 156, 198; Sleazy Surgeon, 72, 74, 80, 87–91, 164–65
Certitude. *See* Surgical temperament
Changing attitudes toward doctors: nurses', 73, 196; patients', 192–99
Changing medicine and surgery, 150–51, 183–209. *See also* "Old days," the
Character, 10, 19, 21, 24, 30–32, 65, 126. *See also* Defects, or character flaws

275